# FITNESS SUTRA

## ELIMINATE YOUR LOW BACK PAIN

Treatment & Prevention
without Drugs, Surgery, or Chiropractic Sessions

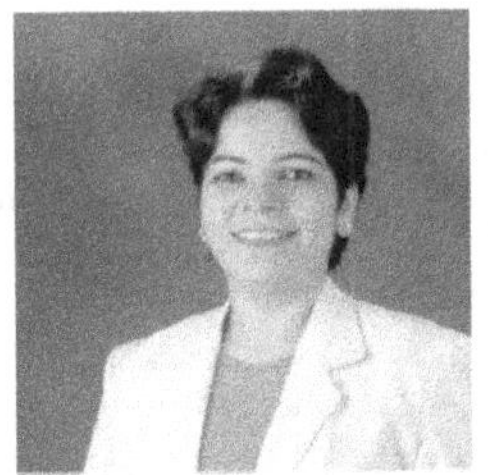

Dr. Monika Chopra
www.fitness-sutra.com

# Dr. Monika Chopra's Fitness Sutra



Published by FitSutra Wellness Pvt Ltd,
33, Prachi Residency, Baner Rd., Pune-411045, India

ISBN-13: 978-1-6738-3232-7



Although I am a Physiotherapist (PT, for those of you in the USA) and a trained Yoga teacher, my suggestions through this book do not establish a doctor-patient relationship between us. This book is not intended to be a substitute for the medical advice of physicians. You should regularly consult a physician in matters relating to your health particularly with respect to any symptoms that may require diagnosis or medical attention. I advise you to take full responsibility of your safety and be aware of your physical limits. Before practising the exercises described in this book, be sure that your equipment is well maintained. Do not take risks beyond your level of flexibility, aptitude, strength, and comfort level.

This is a work of nonfiction. No names have been changed, no characters invented and no events fabricated. The information provided within this Book is for general informational purposes only. While I have tried to keep the information up-to-date and correct, there are no representations or warranties, expressed or implied, about the completeness, accuracy, reliability, suitability or availability with respect to the information, products, services, or related graphics contained in this book for any purpose. Any use of this information is at the reader's own responsibility. I do not assume and hereby disclaim any liability to any party for any loss, damage, or disruption caused by errors or omissions, whether such errors or omissions result from negligence, accident, or any other cause.

# What to Expect from this Book?

Today low back pain has become one of the most common causes of disability in young and adults. Often it impacts everything in your life from sitting to driving, standing, walking, spending time with your loved ones, doing laundry and kitchen work, engaging in recreational activities, sports and the list continues

At times you get frustrated trying to calm down the pain through various available methods. You need a road map to help to navigate through all the potential problems and what to do about them.

This book is for everyone who is currently suffering from low back ache or has suffered it in the past. It is also for those who want to prevent themselves from low back ache and aim for an active, pain free life.

This book is a step by step guide to understanding the problem and providing a real life solution for low back pain. Through this book, I will teach you which movements and positions can cause you pain and which ones can alleviate pain. I will guide you to what remedies can be started immediately at home to decrease the pain, including hot/cold treatments, Myofascial Release (MFR), strengthening and stretching exercises. I will also give you ergonomic tips on how to protect your back while sitting, standing, lifting objects, lying down, driving etc. thus preventing the onset of low back pain in future.

This book will help you to understand what is going on in your body that is causing so much pain. You can work towards designing the right pain relief plan and be empowered to treat yourself.

# CONTENTS

# CHAPTER 1

## Introduction to Low Back Pain

If you have low back pain you are not alone. About 80% of adults experience Low Back Pain (LBP) at some point in their lifetime. LBP can impact everything in your life from walking to driving, even just sitting at your desk can cause extreme pain. It is the most common cause of job related disability and a leading contributor to missed work days.

### *Who Are Prone To Low Back Aches*

Men and women are equally affected by LBP, which can range in intensity from a dull, constant ache to a sudden, sharp sensation that leaves one incapacitated. Onset of pain can be sudden, as a result of an accident or by lifting, pulling or pushing something heavy, or it can develop over time due to age-related changes of spine. Sedentary lifestyles can also lead to LBP, especially when a weekday's routine of getting too little exercise is punctuated by strenuous weekend workout. Driving or sitting in hunched position, bending awkwardly or being in this position for long periods of time are common causes of LBP. Overweight people, smokers, pregnant females, stressed or depressed people; people on long term use of medicines that weaken bones e.g. corticosteroids and those leading sedentary lifestyle are more at risk of low back pain.

*Classification of Low Back Pain on Basis of Duration of its Existence*

1. <u>Acute or Short Term Low Back Pain</u>: Acute low back pain lasts for a few days or a few weeks. It tends to resolve on its own with self-care and there is no residual loss of function. The majority of low back pain is mechanical in nature, i.e. there is a disruption in the way the components of the back (i.e. spine, muscles, intervertebral discs and nerves) fit together and move.

2. <u>Sub-acute Low Back Pain</u>: When the low back pain persists for six weeks to three months it is known as sub-acute low back pain. This type of pain is usually mechanical in nature (such as a muscle or joint pain), but is prolonged. A medical checkup should be considered and is advisable if the pain is severe and limits one's ability to participate in activities of daily living, sleeping and working.

3. <u>Chronic Low Back Pain</u>: Low back pain that lasts over three months is considered as chronic low back pain. This type of pain is usually severe, does not respond to initial treatments and requires a thorough medical investigation to determine the exact source of the pain.

# CHAPTER 2

## Muscles that Support your Lower Back – How their Weakness or Tightness can lead to Low Back Pain

The lower back supports the weight of upper body and provides mobility for the everyday movements including bending and twisting. The muscles in the lower back are responsible for flexing, extending and rotating the hips while walking as well as supporting the spinal column. Nerves in the low back supply sensation and power to the muscles in the pelvis, legs, and feet.

Most acute and chronic low back pain results from injury to muscles, ligaments, joints, discs or nerve involvement.

*Muscles Supporting Low Back and their Function*

Soft tissues around the spine play a key role in low back. These are a large and complex group of muscles that work together to support the spine and help in

- Flexion (bending forward)
- Extension (bending backwards)
- Side flexion (side bending) and
- Rotation movement at the spine.

1. <u>Flexor Muscles</u> that are attached to the front of spine enable forward bending (flexion), lifting and arching of lower back.

2. <u>Extensor Muscles</u> that are attached to the back of the spine enable standing and lifting objects. These muscles include mainly erector spinae (which helps in holding up the spine) and gluteal muscles (hip muscles).

3. <u>Oblique Muscles</u> that are attached to the sides of the spine, help rotate the spine.

4. Along with the above mentioned muscles, there are hip flexors (muscles present in front of the hip joint) and hip extensors (especially hamstrings) present behind hip joint.

5. The large muscles present in the back of the thighs, play an important role in supporting the spine.

*Effect of Altered Muscle Strength and Flexibility on Low Back*

Muscle strength and flexibility are essential to maintain spine in neutral position. Muscle strength and flexibility can be affected in the following ways, leading to low back pain.

1. Deep back muscles and abdominal muscles tend to weaken with age if not specially exercised. Weak abdominal muscles cause hip flexors to tighten thus causing an increase in the lower back curve (*hyperlordosis* or swayback). This leads to an unhealthy posture thus causing low back pain.

2.  Inflammation or injury in or around the spine causes large back muscles to go in spasm thus leading to lower back pain and marked movement limitations.

3.  Disuse of muscles during an episode of prolonged low back pain (more than 2-3 weeks) can lead to muscle weakness which in turn leads to low back pain because weakened muscles are not able to support the spine.

4.  Stress can lead to muscle weakness and back pain. When stressed, back muscles become tight in fight or flight response leading to pains & spine inflexibility and increase the risk of spinal injury. Chronic unmanaged stress, experienced daily and repeated over weeks, months or even years, can virtually cripple your back by causing devastating chronic muscle tension that distorts the normal alignment of the spine.

5.  Tight hamstring muscles can also cause low back pain.

Strengthening and stretching exercises specific to abdominal muscles, back muscles, hamstrings and hip flexor muscles, as mentioned in upcoming chapters, help to treat back pain by reinforcing support to the spine. Regular & correct exercising may even eliminate the need of surgery.

*Understand Your Core – It's Importance for a Pain Free Back*

Core of the body is broadly the torso of the body. Core muscles work together to give maximum stability to lumbar (low back) and abdominal region, as well as coordinate movements of legs, arms and spine. Major Core muscles include transverse abdominis muscle, multifidus, erector spinae, diaphragm, external and internal obliques and pelvic floor muscles.

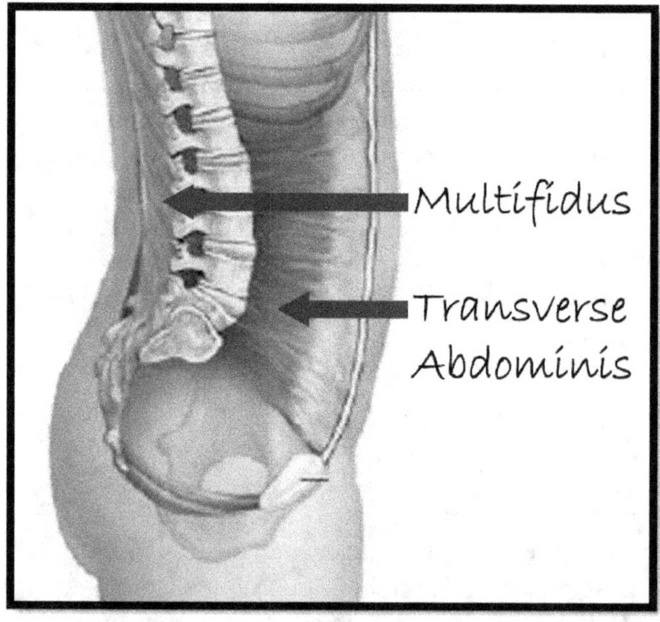


Low back pain can be triggered by a number of reasons like muscle strain, muscle overuse and injuries to muscles, ligaments or discs that support spine.

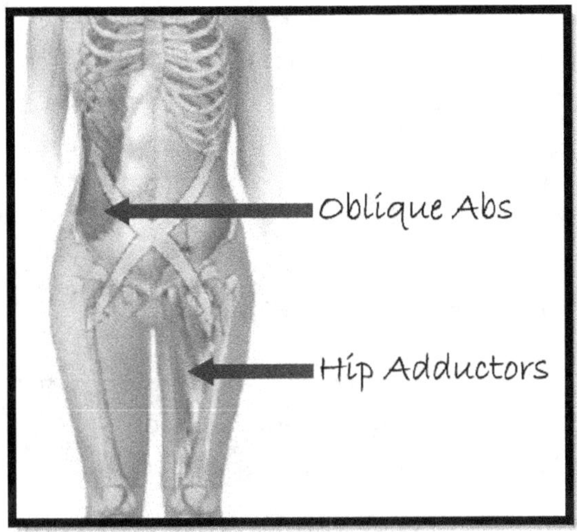


Over course of time the injury in or around the spine, if not taken care of, can lead to overall imbalances in the spine. This can lead to constant tension or weakness in muscles, ligaments and bones, making the back more prone to injury and re-injury.

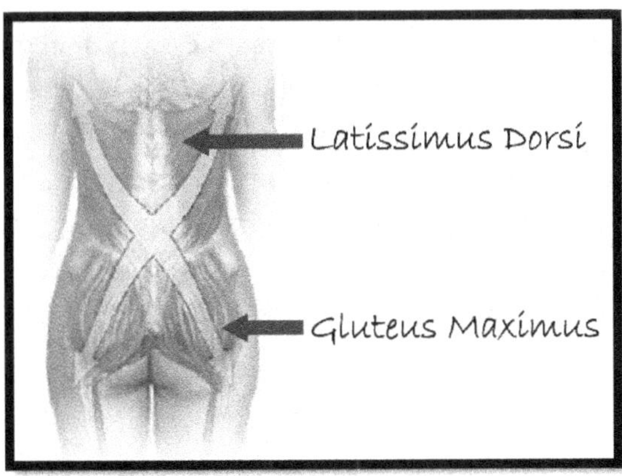

Rehabilitation programs or preventive rehabilitation programs that focus on strengthening lumbar muscles combined with core stability and proprioception help in reducing the risk of low back pain if exercises are done correctly and on regular basis.

## *Where and How to Palpate Core Muscles*

It is important to understand how and where you feel the core muscles working when you do core strengthening and stability exercises.

In order to understand that you are contracting correct muscles, it is important to learn how to feel them contracting. Place your hand on the bony parts at front of your hips. These are known as *Anterior Superior Iliac Spine* (ASIS). Move your hand in an inch towards your belly button and down an inch towards your toes. You should now be directly above transverse abdominis muscle.

When all the core muscles co-contract you will feel gentle tightening of transverse muscle too. If you feel a bulge, you are contracting core muscles too strong. The correct level of activity in core muscles should be 30% of the maximum contract level so that you can keep on contracting these muscles continuously.

# Bonus

I hope you are finding this book useful and are ready to start with the exercises.

I have also created an easy to use quick reference chart of these exercises. Placed at a prominent place in your bedroom, this would serve as a handy reminder to do your exercises at regular interval.

You can download the printable file from

**https://www.fitness-sutra.com/go?id=141004**

You can also subscribe to my mailing list to get more tips & motivation to do these exercises.

# CHAPTER 3

## Anatomy of Spine

Proper treatment of any condition starts with the education of the condition. In my experience as a medical professional, first few appointments in clinical setting go to the proper understanding of the problem and how it can be managed. With good understanding of the situation, you can comprehend and follow the treatment plan better.

In order to explain the cause of low back pain, I will start with some basic anatomy of the back (especially spine and back muscles) and then move into more specifics.

### General Anatomy of Spine

Our spine is made up of a large stack of bones called vertebrae, which are separated by strong cushions called inter-vertebral discs. The vertebrae are labelled by section from top to bottom. In the neck, they are called cervical vertebrae and are labelled "C1" to "C7" (collectively called Cervical Spine). Below the neck, they are called thoracic vertebrae and are labelled "T1" to "T12" (collectively called Thoracic Spine). This is your upper/middle back. Finally in the low back they are called lumbar vertebrae and labelled "L1" to "L5" (collectively called Lumbar Spine). Below the lumbar vertebrae is a large bone called the sacrum which is referred to as "S".

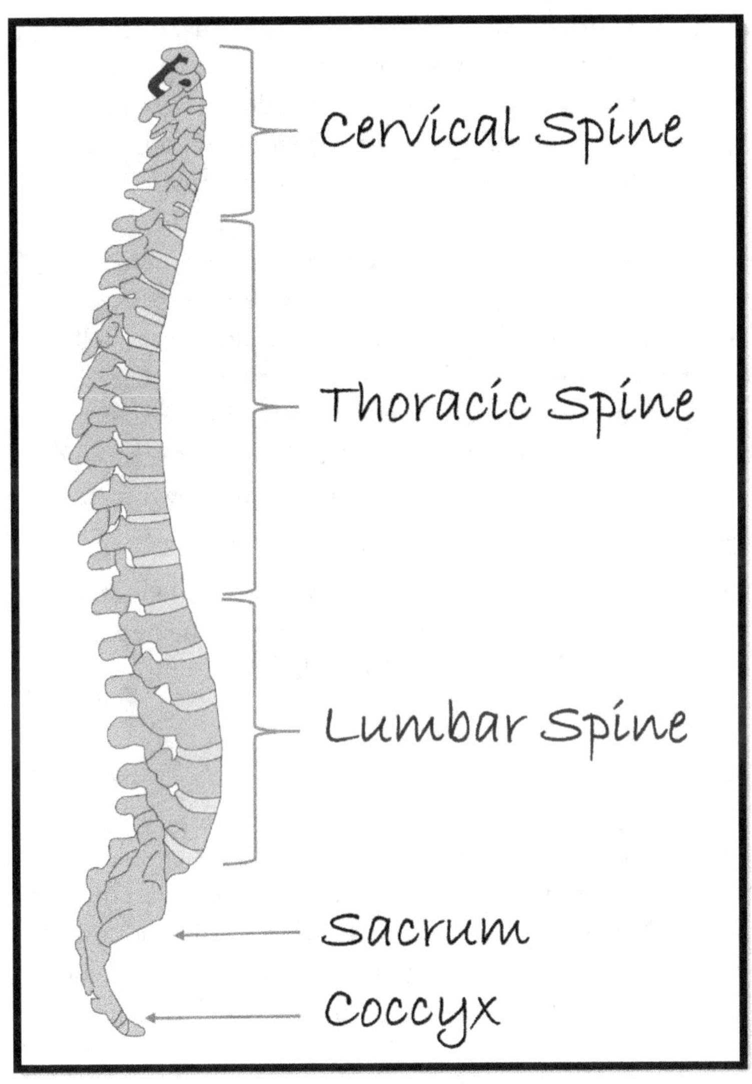


A healthy spine is important to maintain the balance of the whole body during movement and rest.

The spinal cord passes through the spinal canal of the vertebrae. Between the vertebrae there are nerves that extend off the spinal cord in each direction. These nerves travel on a very specific path through the body and are responsible for controlling pain, sensation, muscle response and reflexes in those areas. The path for each nerve has been mapped and is common for all men & women. According to the area where you are experiencing pain, weakness or other symptoms, your doctor can tell which nerve might be affected. For example, the nerves exiting from the area in the neck go down in a specific pattern to arms. The nerves of the mid back wrap around the ribs. And the nerves of low back extend down to the legs.

The nerves are labelled by stating the level of the vertebrae above and below where the nerve exits. E.g. the nerve that exits below "L3" and above "L4" is labelled as "L3-L4".

*The Lumbo-Sacral Complex*

The lumbo-sacral complex is an important functional unit of the body consisting of five lumbar vertebrae and the sacrum. The lumbar spine starts below the ribs and ends in sacrum which is next to the pelvis. The lumbar vertebrae, because of their weight bearing function, are large and massive.

At each level of the lumbar spine there is a nerve that exits. These nerves branch out and extend down to different areas in our legs and feet. Each nerve has a specific pattern and is responsible for control of specific muscles as well as control of specific reflexes. By identifying the area of pain, muscle weakness and reflexes involved we can determine which nerve is involved.

As the nerve exits the spine it first goes through a small hole called *neural foramen*. The space within the foramina is particularly important. If it is smaller than normal, then it can cause pain and weakness anywhere along the path that the specific nerve travels. The foramina is particularly vulnerable for impingement of the emerging spinal nerves by tumor, trauma or degenerative changes. Among degenerative changes, osteoarthritis is a common cause where small uneven calcium deposits form on the inside of the hole making it smaller over time.

*The Intervertebral Disc*

An intervertebral disc is a pad between each vertebrae in our spine. The discs act as shock absorbers of the spine. They hold the vertebrae together and allow slight movement of the vertebrae which helps in movement of rotation and bending. Discs help to cushion weight and sheer forces on the back while maintaining space between the vertebras so that the peripheral nerves (reaching various parts of the body) get space to exit from the central nervous system.

## Structure of a Disc

The disc can be compared to a donut filled with jelly where jelly represents *nucleus pulposus* and donut represents *annulus fibrosis.*

The gelatinous material of nucleus pulposus is normally under considerable pressure. This is prevented to go out of the disc by the concentric *fibro-cartilaginous* rings of annulus fibrosis.

## Prolapsed Intervertebral Disc

There are various lesions that can occur in an intervertebral disc. The most common are extrusion (herniated disc) and protrusion (bulging disc).

## Disc Protrusion (Bulging Disc)

Under pressure, the nucleus fluid may sometimes bulge out through weakened areas of annulus. This is called protrusion. The increased pressure can be from lifting something heavy, poor posture while sitting etc. Often times, this happens over several years as some of the fibrous layers of annulus start to break leaving a weak spot in the disc. Most of the time the disc bulges more to one side than another and the symptoms related to nerve compression of that side occur (eg. pain down one leg along with back pain). But sometimes the disc bulge can be central, thus putting pressure on the spinal cord and thereby producing symptoms related to that (eg. radiating pain in both legs along with back ache).

Mostly by good management (exercises) and sensible lifestyle, one can get full pain free function after protrusion. However for patients with higher disc vulnerability and persistent episodic pain, surgical intervention is justified.

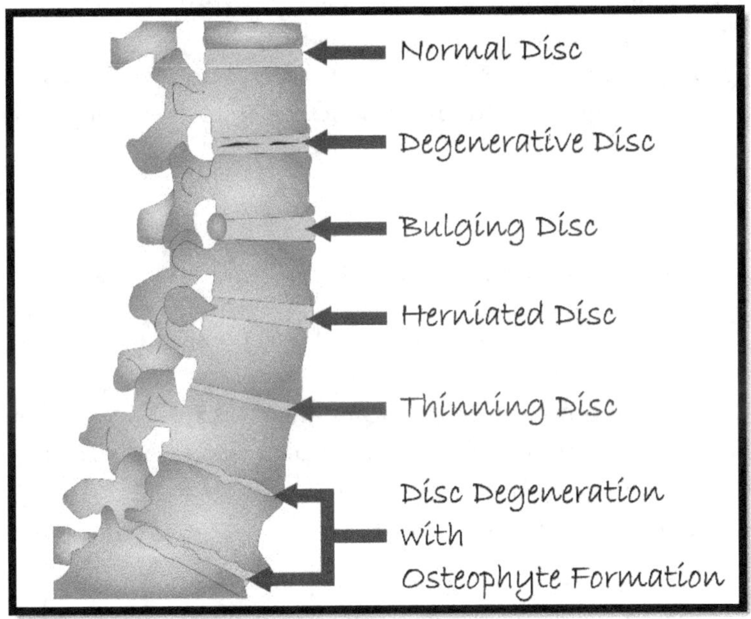


*Extrusion (Herniated Disc)*

A split may occur in annulus fibrosis and since the nucleus pulposus is under pressure, fluid moves into the split. The nucleus may extrude centrally backwards into the spinal canal causing damage to the nerve roots, nerves, ligaments around it etc.

In most of the minor cases, the fibrous tissue can close the split in annulus and thus repair occurs. Yet, the healed area may remain weak and thus become prone to further lesions unless a strict program for spinal care is followed. The extruded nuclear fluid is replaced by fibrous tissue which shrinks. This may cause adhesions between the ligaments, nerve roots, spine and vertebrae and result in persistent pain if no attempt is made to restore mobility of tissue.

*Symptoms of Lumbar Herniated Disc*

The symptoms of lumbar herniated disc may vary from moderate pain in back and buttocks to widespread weakness and numbness requiring medical care. Disc herniation is often times more painful at the onset because of the inflammatory changes around the surrounding nerves due to leaked out gel.

1. <u>Low back pain:</u> A dull throbbing low back pain associated with low back muscle spasm may occur due to disc herniation. One can feel low back stiffness. Normally this pain and stiffness can be alleviated somewhat by one or two days' rest, ice and heat treatment of low back, sitting in a reclined

supported position or lying flat on the back with knees slightly flexed and supported on pillow.

2. <u>Leg pain</u>: Leg pain may be more severe than low back pain as the herniated disc puts pressure on the nerve root innervating the legs. The pain that radiates along the path of the sciatic nerve to the back of the leg is commonly referred to as sciatica or radiculopathy. The nerve pain can be described as sharp, searing, stabbing, electric, radiating or piercing.

3. <u>Neurological symptoms</u>: Symptoms like numbness, pins and needles feeling, weakness and tingling sensation may be present in the nerve root distribution in leg, feet or toes.

4. <u>Variable location of symptoms</u>: Depending on the variables like where the disc is herniated and degree of herniation; symptoms may be experienced in low back, buttocks, front and back of thighs, calves, feet or toes. It typically affects just one side of the body.

5. <u>Foot drop</u>: Foot drop is difficulty in lifting the foot when walking or standing on the ball of the foot. This may occur if disc herniation affects the nerve supplying foot.

6. <u>Pain that worsens with the movement</u>: Pain may occur after prolonged sitting, standing or after

short distance walking. Any sudden action like laughing, sneezing, coughing or bowel movement may intensify the pain.

As mentioned earlier, the fibrous tissue can close the split in annulus leading to repair in majority of the cases, thus the pain may ease within six weeks' time.

*Risk Factors for Lumbar Disc Herniation*

1. <u>Age</u>:  This most commonly affects people between ages 20-55 years. It can occur in older people too.

2. <u>Gender</u>: Men have roughly twice the risk for lumbar disc herniation compared to women. It's because this damage is related to heavy, repeated work more commonly undertaken by males than females.

3. <u>Sites</u>: Most commonly affected sites are "L5-S" and "L4-L5", but all lumbar discs are prone to prolapse.

4. <u>Physically demanding work</u>: Jobs that require heavy lifting, repeated pulling, pushing and twisting action and other physical labor are more prone to lumbar disc herniation.

5. <u>Obesity</u>: Excess weight increases the chances of lumbar disc herniation and twelve times more

chance of recurrent disc herniation (i.e. herniation of same disc again) after a micro-discectomy surgery. Being overweight or obese adds to the stress being placed on the spinal discs, accelerating their breakdown and hence leading to lumbar disc herniation.

6. <u>Smoking</u>: Nicotine decreases the blood flow to the spinal discs thus accelerating disc degeneration and hampering it's healing. Degenerated discs are less pliable and more prone to wear and tear thus leading to disc herniation.

7. <u>Family history</u>: There are medical records of hereditary tendency for disc degeneration and lumbar disc herniation. Studies show that family history of lumbar disc herniation can predict the occurrence of future lumbar disc herniation.

Though above factors increase the risk of lumbar disc herniation, it is possible for an individual of any age and gender to have a lumbar disc herniation. At times, it may occur for no known reasons.

# CHAPTER 4

## First Aid for Low Back Pain

Self-care for low back pain (acute or chronic) can be started at home before visiting a doctor or therapist. It includes basic techniques like rest, hot and cold treatment, posture correction, stretching and strengthening exercises and over the counter medicines (OTC). The correct understanding of how and when these various techniques should be applied is important to get the desired result.

In this chapter, I will be giving you an insight of how and when various self-care techniques can be applied and what impact they have on the paining back.

*Short Period Rest*

Rest helps to reduce the back pain by decreasing the pressure on the intervertebral discs and also by decreasing the mechanical stresses that may be irritating the pain receptors. Though 1-2 days of rest is advisable, more than this can be detrimental to the recovery. Too much bed rest can lead to muscle atrophy, cardio-pulmonary deconditioning, an illness mindset, bone mineral loss and in some cases even blood clots.

The appropriate way to lie down during bed rest is in side lying with upper leg and arm supported on pillows, parallel to the lying down surface, maintaining the natural spinal curves.

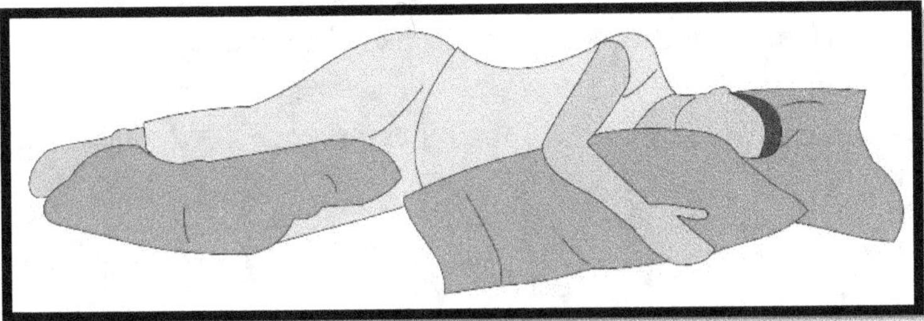

If lying on back, try to maintain the lumbar curve by inserting a small rolled towel behind low back, keeping knees slightly bent.

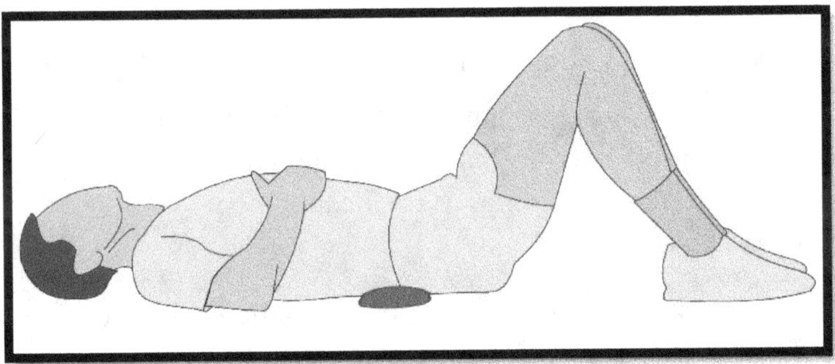

## Activity Modification

A very good way of staying active and also avoiding low back pain is by doing activities and getting into postures that do not aggravate the pain. For example, if sitting for long hours (e.g. sitting in the office or driving) increases the pain, you can take standing or walking breaks or even do back stretches every 20 minutes. This helps to break the buildup of stress in the back muscles and thus prevents them from going into spasm which lead to back pain. If standing for long hours (doing house chores etc.) is straining the back, you can sit or lie down or do stretches to decrease the stress and thus relieve pain.

*Heat Therapy*

Heat therapy provides pain relief as well as healing benefit in low back pain. Heat therapy can be given with hot water bottle, electric heating pads, warm baths or chemical or adhesive heat wraps.

How heat therapy works: Heating dilates the blood vessels of the muscles surrounding the spine. This leads to increased blood flow in this area bringing more nutrients and oxygen, thus speeding up the healing process of damaged tissues.

Heat stimulates the sensory receptors of the skin which diminishes the pain sensation signals reaching the brain, thus decreasing the pain perception and discomfort.

Heat therapy improves the flexibility of muscles and connective tissues surrounding the spine. With decreased stiffness, the chances of injury to the spine decreases. Increased flexibility makes the spine movements more comfortable.

Why Heat Therapy? The plus point of Heat therapy is that it is an inexpensive mode of treatment (You can have it while taking hot water bath).  It can be applied anywhere. You can use a hot water bottle while lying down or while sitting you can put hot packs behind your back etc. Portable heating wraps can be carried to the work or while traveling and can be used while sitting. Being a non-invasive and non-medicinal form of treatment, heat therapy is preferred by many. It can be used with other physiotherapy modalities like TENS, to give quicker results.

How much heat should be applied to body? The temperature of the heating source should be enough to reach the muscles. 'Warm' is good as it can reach the muscles deeply without burning the skin. 'Too Hot' temperature can be uncomfortable to bear and 'Slightly Warm' may not reach the deeper muscle layers. The duration of heat application to the affected area depends on the kind of injury. For small tension or little back pain, 15 to 20 minutes of heat application should be good enough to relieve pain. For acute and chronic pain, this duration can be increased to 30 minutes to 2 hours.

Types of Heat Therapy: There are two types of heat therapies – Moist Heat Therapy and Dry Heat Therapy. Moist heat (e.g. hot bath, moist heating packs and moist towel) makes the area suppler and some people find it better than Dry heat (e.g. electric heating pads, hot water bottle and sauna) which heats the body part but makes it dry. Some people prefer Dry heat as it is easier to apply.

<u>Various ways of Heat application:</u>

1. <u>Hot Bath, Hot Tubs, Steam Baths & Sauna</u>: This gives a general feeling of relaxation to the body thus reducing muscle spasm and pain. A whirlpool jet directed to a specific part of the body has an added benefit of localized light massage.
2. <u>Hot Water Bottle</u>: This is one of the easiest ways of applying heat to any localized area of body. It stays warm for good 15-20 minutes and can be applied sitting and lying down.
3. <u>Electric Heating Pads</u>: This is also a very easy and less cumbersome way of applying heat. The electric heating pad provides a constant heat till the pad is plugged to the source.
4. <u>Heating Gel Packs</u>: These can be heated in microwave or by putting in hot water. The gel remains warm for 25-30 minutes. Some gel packs also give moist heat.
5. <u>Heat Wraps</u>: The best part of this heating technique is that it can be applied to the skin, under your clothing and you can move around with it or can carry it anywhere. It stays warm for longer duration.

Heat therapy can be applied to local, regional or whole body. For local area, small heat gel packs or hot water bottle works well. Regional treatment works well for more widespread area of pain and stiffness. Heat wraps, hot water towel and large sized heat pads work well for this.

For full body treatment, sauna bath and hot tub is preferable.

<u>Things to consider before using Heat Therapy</u>: Heat therapy should not be applied if the lower back is swollen or bruised. In case of heart disease or hypertension, consult your doctor before heat application. Pregnant females should avoid hot tub or sauna bath.

Few conditions where heat therapy cannot be used are:

- Sensory changes – Can't feel if it is too hot.
- Circulatory problems.
- During acute phase of injury (area is swollen or bruised)
- Deep vein thrombosis (DVT)
- Infections
- Malignant tumor
- Hyper or Hypo sensitivity
- Diabetes
- Peripheral vascular disease
- Severe cognitive impairment
- Dermatitis
- Multiple sclerosis

The heat therapy increases the flow of blood in the particular area. In conditions such as circulatory problems, DVT, peripheral vascular disease, regulation of blood flow is an issue. In conditions such as infections or malignant tumors, the enhanced blood flow increases the chances of spread of infection or cancerous cells.

<u>Warning</u>: If there is an increase in the swelling of the area due to heat application, immediately stop heat therapy. In case heat therapy is not reducing the pain or stiffness, consult your doctor.

## *Cold / Cryotherapy*

Cryotherapy is a simple and effective technique which reduces muscle spasm and inflammation in acute phase of injury. It is most beneficial when used within 24 to 48 hours of injury. It is one of the best pain management techniques immediately after the onset of muscle spasm.

In most of the cases the cause of sudden low back pain is the muscle strain which can occur due to poor posture, sudden bending and lifting of heavy loads, twisting, sudden fall, getting into an awkward position which causes back strain or sports related injury. Applying ice along with short period of rest, pain medications and taking anti-inflammatory drugs, can relieve one from this kind of pain.

<u>How Icing Works</u>: Icing constrict the blood vessels thus reducing the blood flow in the area where it is applied. This decreases the swelling and inflammation in the affected area. Once the cold application is removed, the blood vessels compensate by over-dilating and thus blood rushes into the area. The infusion of blood in the area brings along with it nutrients, which aid in healing of injured back muscles, ligaments and tendons.

Icing can temporarily reduce the nerve activity, which can also relieve pain. Icing decreases the tissue damage. Ice massage adds to the effect by providing soft tissue manipulation.

<u>Techniques of Using Cryotherapy</u>: The patient should sit or lie down in a comfortable position. To cover the lower back, lying on abdomen with hips slightly flexed (you can place a small pillow under the hips) is the best position as it decreases strain on low back.

<u>Various ways of Cold Therapy</u>:

1. <u>Ice Packs or Frozen Gel Packs</u>. Many types of ice packs or ice gel packs are available in the market. These can be used directly on the pain area or you can wrap it in a towel and place on injured part. A duration of 15 to 20 minutes of ice pack application is good enough to get the desired effect. It can be used 8-10 times a day.

2. <u>Reusable Ice Packs</u>: Many types of reusable ice packs are available in the drug stores or merchandise stores. You can keep them in your refrigerator and can use when required. These can be frozen in the refrigerator for a number of times. They are easy to use and are relatively inexpensive.

3. <u>Disposable / Instant Ice Packs</u>: These are instant ice packs which become cold immediately after the seal is opened (chemical reaction occurs in the pack when it is opened). The plus point of these packs is that they are ready to use when required as prior cooling is not essential. Since the cooling

happens because of the chemical reaction happening in the pack, they stay cooler for longer hours at room temperature.

4. <u>Homemade Ice Packs</u>: You can make your own ice packs with material available in home. You can freeze a wet fluffy towel, wet sponge, some rice in socks, some water in a plastic bag or simply grab a packet of frozen food and place on the affected area. You can roll the uneven food packet in a light towel to increase its effectiveness.

5. <u>Ice Massage</u>. You can use ice directly on the affected area by moving it in a circular motion for not more than 2-3 minutes. A maximum of 5-6 sq inch area should be covered at a time. The direct application of ice numbs the painful area instantly and circular massaging movement relaxes the strained area. Ice massage can be repeated 4-5 times in a day.

6. <u>Ice Baths</u>: Ice bath (4-5 minutes application on affected area) is effective in reduction of acute and chronic back pain.

<u>Things to consider before using Cold Therapy</u>: Few conditions where cold therapy cannot be used are:

- Rheumatoid arthritis
- Hypertension
- History of vascular impairment (frostbite or atherosclerosis)
- Local limb ischemia

- Raynaud's syndrome
- Cold allergic conditions
- Impaired sensory sensations
- Paralysis

<u>Warning</u>: Direct application of ice can cause ice burns. Keep moving the ice during ice massage. Never sleep with ice on your skin.

## Use of Back Brace

Many types of back braces are available in the market. For low back pain lumbar back brace is the best. Back brace provides extra support to your lower back bones and muscles and limits the movement in the back, thus relieving the pain.

Too much use of back braces should be avoided as it can weaken the muscles and ligaments of that area, thus making spine prone to injuries.

## Over The Counter Medications (OTC)

Most commonly used OTC medications are:

- Pain Killers: E.g. Acetaminophen (Tylenol). Acetaminophen works by blocking the pain signals sent to brain.
- NSAIDS (Non-Steroidal Anti-Inflammatory Drugs): E.g. Aspirin, Ibuprofen, Naproxen. These

alleviate the pain by reducing the inflammation of swollen nerves and muscles.

<u>Note</u>: Normally self-care with OTC drugs can be done without doctor's advice. But as with any other medication or treatment, above mentioned treatments and medications may be associated with some side effects. In case the above mentioned treatments do not bring relief for a week or you see any side effects, please consult your doctor immediately.

# CHAPTER 5

## Myofascial Release

Majority of low back pain cases are an outcome of the lifestyle issues. Prolonged sitting, wrong working posture, performing repetitive tasks (as in a sedentary lifestyle) can exacerbate the pain. These habits decrease the spinal mobility, increase muscle stress and thus spasm and lead to weakness of the muscles. The most commonly involved muscles are core muscles and hip flexor and extensor muscles. By doing stretching, strengthening and mobility exercises targeting these muscles, one can get rid of low back pain in most of the cases.

Another important factor in structural integrity of spine is the fascia. Fascia is a sheet of connective tissue beneath the skin that attaches, stabilizes, encloses and separates muscles, bones and other internal organs. It plays an important role in maintaining postural alignment and ease of movement. Poor lifestyle habits, posture and movement patterns can lead to stiffness of fascia, thus restricting movements and causing pain. By proper myofascial techniques the flexibility of fascia can be maintained.

In this chapter we will discuss the myofascial techniques, stretching, strengthening and mobility exercises of mainly core muscles, glutes, hamstring and piriformis muscles, which can bring relief from back pain without getting into invasive surgeries and popping medicines.

Myofascial release exercises work as deep tissue massage to tight muscles and fascia (*Trigger Points*), loosening them, so that the stretches are more effective. Trigger points are specific spots in muscles (also referred to as '*knots*') where muscles have decreased blood circulation, increased contraction and a build-up of toxic waste. A trigger point can exist in two states

- Active trigger point – This is very painful as you touch on it or around it.
- Latent trigger point – This is typically pain free unless touched hard or poked in it.

Here we are going to target following main muscles –

1. Gluteus Maximus: Gluteus maximus is the main extensor of hip. It is the biggest of gluteus muscles and one of the main trigger points for pain.

2. Gluteus Medius and Minimus: The Gluteus Medius is a thick fan shaped muscle lying over the smaller Gluteus Minimus and underneath the larger Gluteus Maximus muscle. The primary function of the Gluteus Medius is shared with the Gluteus Minimus and that is to abduct the thigh at the hips, and laterally rotating the thigh at the hips as well as stabilizing the body when one foot is raised off the ground during walking and running. Trigger points in these muscles may cause low back pain.

3.  <u>Piriformis:</u> Piriformis lies deep under gluteus muscle. It runs from back of femur (thigh bone) to sacrum (base of the spine). Tightness in this muscle can be related to sacroiliac joint dysfunction and also sciatica like pain.

We would use a moderately firm ball (like a lacrosse or tennis ball) for precise targeting of trigger points. Some Important tips for myofascial release are:

- Warm the hip first with light exercises or heating pad.
- When you find the tender spot, hold the ball there for 20 seconds. The pressure there should cause release of tension with 'happy pain' making the area relax and increase flexibility.
- Breathe deeply into the relaxing muscle.
- The pain due to the exercise should be dull 'happy pain'. If the pain is sharp shooting pain, immediately stop the exercise.
- Do static stretching of the area afterwards.

*Gluteus Maximus Myofascial Release*

The gluteus maximus is the large muscle group that forms the buttocks.

- The medial trigger point is found adjacent to the lower sacrum, near the muscle's medial attachment.

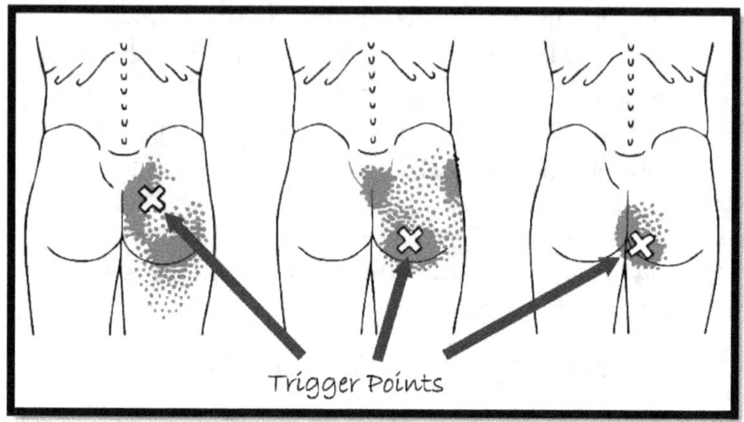



- The other two trigger points in this muscle appear lower, one lies near the ischial tuberosity and one lies on the inside edge of the gluteal fold region, below the tailbone or coccyx.

*Myofascial Release Technique of Gluteus Maximus*

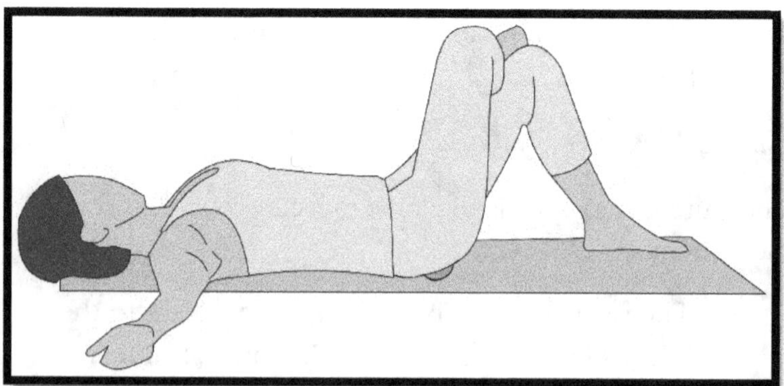

_Start Position:_    Once you have located the muscle, place the ball under it and lie down on your back. Make a figure of 'Four' with your legs, with the leg having tender point resting on the knee of the other leg. In the illustration, the patient is trying to release the pain on right hip.

_Steps:_

1.  The ball can be slid on the gluteal muscle in the above position. As you roll the ball here, you will spot the tender point.
2.  Let the ball be there at the tender point. Enjoy the _'happy pain'_ as you feel the contracted tissues relax.
3.  Try to move the ball to all the tender points mentioned above and relax them.

## _Gluteus Medius & Minimus Myofascial Release_

Gluteus medius and minimus start from top of the hip bone to outside of your thigh bone. They can be located just below the belt on the outer side of hips. These are high up fleshy part, above the bone.

These muscles are responsible for external/internal hip rotation and for stabilising pelvis during running and walking.

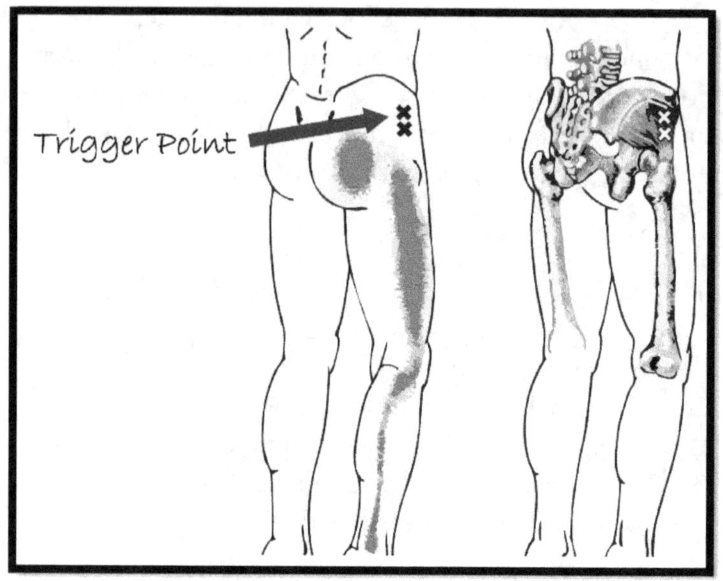


These muscles become tight with muscle work overload during extensive sitting or extensive rotational hip movements. This muscle imbalance can cause pelvis to tilt downward (anterior pelvic tilt), putting excessive pressure on lumbar region, thus causing back pain.

*Myofascial Release Technique of Gluteus Medius and Minimus*

<u>Start Position:</u>    Once you have located the muscle, lie on the side, propped up on your elbow. Flex your lower hip and place the ball on the tender point. The other leg should be flexed and at 90 degrees to the lower leg with knee pointing upwards and upper foot placed flat on floor next to lower leg.

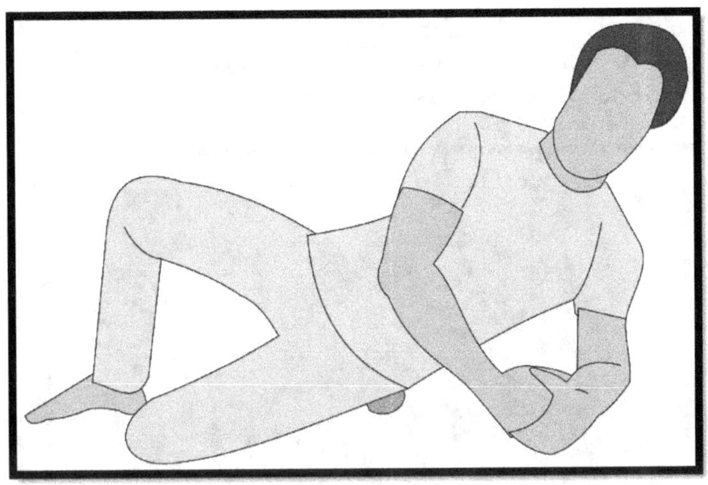

*Steps:*

1.  The ball can be slid on the gluteal muscle in the above position. As you roll the ball here you will find the trigger point.
2.  Let the ball be there at the trigger point.
3.  Enjoy the *'happy pain'* as you feel the contracted tissues relax.

*Fine Tips:*

1.  Maintain a good posture by keeping your shoulders back throughout the release.

*Piriformis Myofascial Release*

Piriformis muscle is located deep beneath the gluteal muscles between sacrum and greater trochanter. To locate the trigger point imagine a line between the sacrum (tail bone) and hip joint and it is present somewhere in mid. It is located deep behind gluteus muscle.

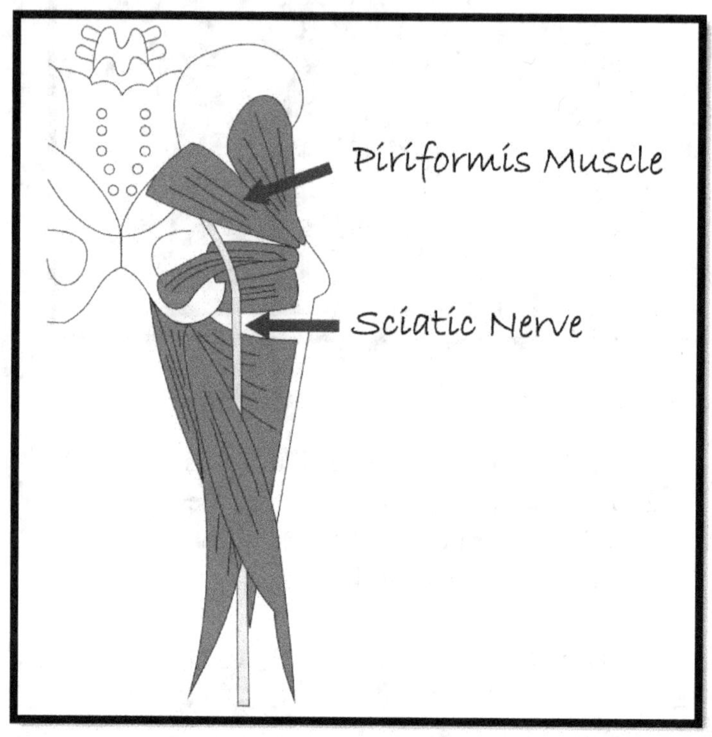


Primary function of piriformis muscle is hip external rotation and abduction. Trigger points can form in piriformis muscle due to overuse (E.g. due to quick changes in direction during sports) or underuse (E.g. due to long hours of sitting). The tight piriformis can lead to impingement of sciatic nerve which can cause pain in lower back, hips and gluteus.

## *Myofascial Release Technique of Piriformis Muscle*

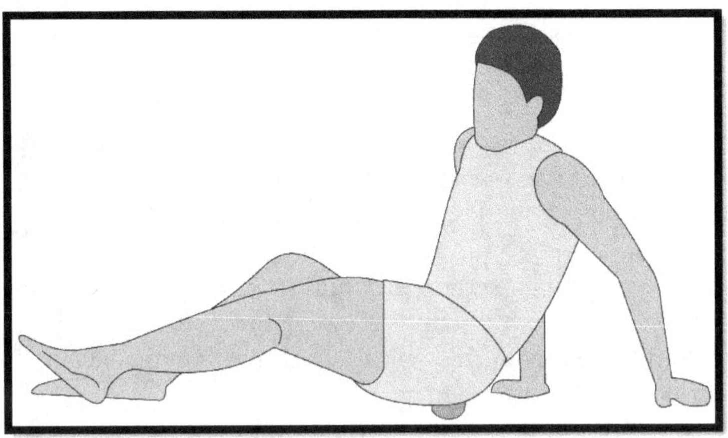

<u>*Start Position:*</u>   Once you have located the piriformis muscle place the ball under it and come in the similar position as for gluteus muscles mentioned above.

<u>*Steps:*</u>

1. Slide the ball little bit in the start position till you find the tender point.
2. Let the ball be there at this point for 20 seconds. Enjoy the 'happy pain' as you feel the contracted tissues relax.
3. As this point relaxes move a little bit towards the sacrum or hip joint. You will find few more tender points. Stretch and relax them the same way.

<u>*Fine Tips:*</u>

1. Maintain a good posture by keeping your shoulders back throughout release.

# CHAPTER 6

## Strengthening Exercises for Back

Low back strengthening and stability exercises can be the best treatment and preventive option for almost all back problems as they tend to restore the balance in the spine.

The strengthening exercise program should be done 3 times a week. The program is divided into 3 levels – easy, medium and difficult. It's important to perfect one level before you move to the next.

Important: The low back pain may occur due to injury to the structures in or around the spine. If the pain is for more than 1-3 weeks, start with the MFR and back pain relieving exercises (see Chapter 10) before moving to strengthening exercises.

# EASY STRENGTHENING EXERCISES FOR BACK

## Pelvic Tilt (Back Imprinting)

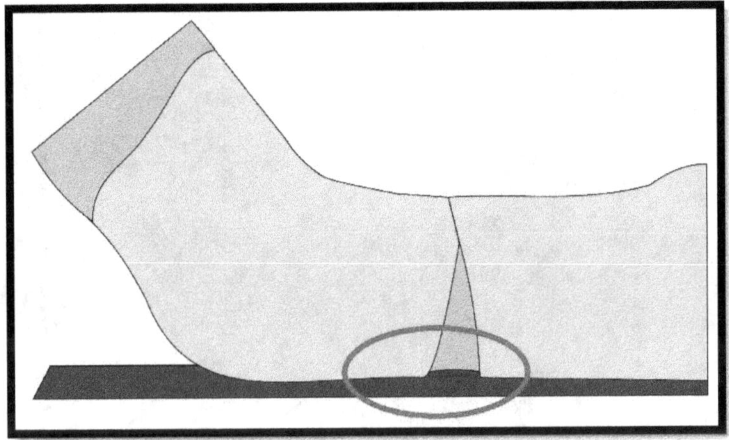

*Start Position:*    Lie down on your back with legs bent, shoulder width apart, feet flat on the mat and arms by the side of your body.

*Steps:*

1. Take your naval in, engaging your abdominal muscles and flatten your lower back on the mat as you exhale.
2. Hold this position as you shallow breathe, for 5 counts.
3. Release the imprint as you inhale.
4. Repeat this sequence 5 times.

## Back Imprinting with One Leg Raise

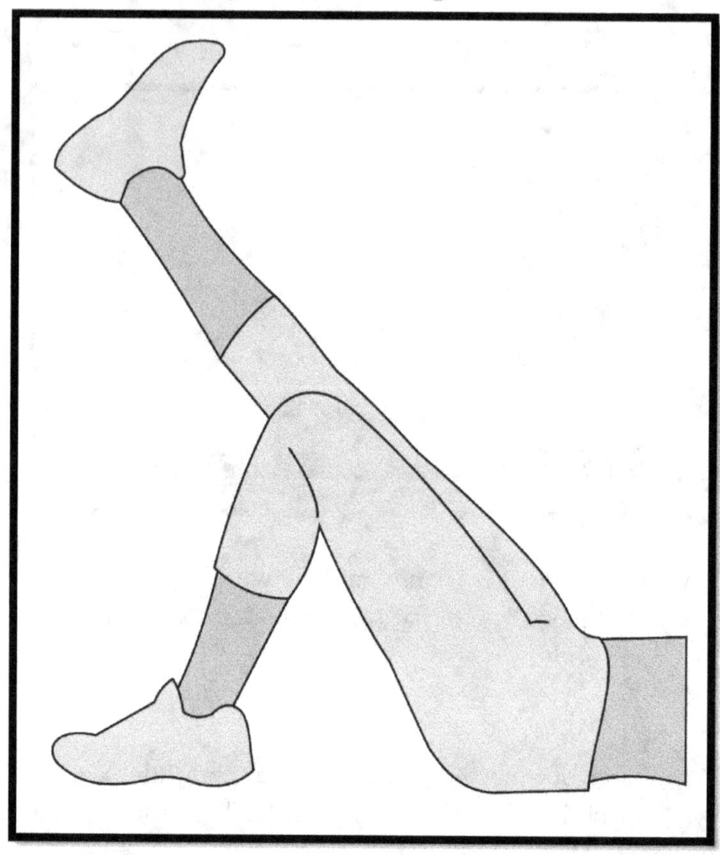

*Effect:*  This exercise helps to strengthen your core muscles along with strengthening of your hip flexors and knee extensors.

*Start Position:*  Lie down on your back with legs bent, shoulder width apart, thigh in line with thigh, feet flat on the mat and arms by the side of your body.

*Steps:*

1. Do back imprinting as mentioned in the earlier exercise.
2. Straighten your right leg at knee, keeping thigh in line with thigh and pull your right foot towards you.
3. Hold this position for 5 counts.
4. Slowly release the imprint and get your right leg back to start position as you inhale.
5. Repeat on the left side.
6. Repeat it 5 times on each side.

## Back Imprinting with One Leg Raise 2"

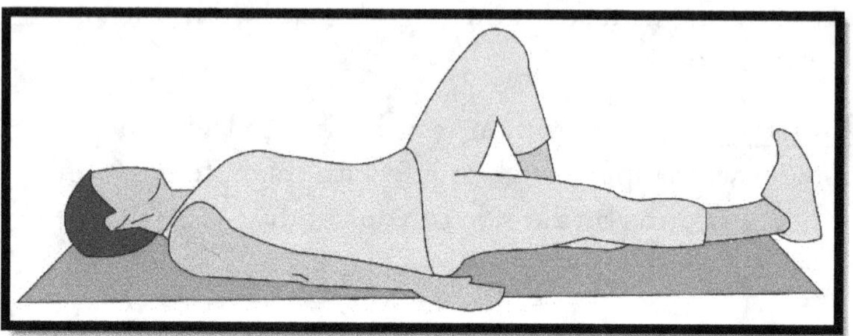

*Effect:*          This is a core strengthening exercise that also strengthens hip flexors.

*Start Position:*   Lie down straight on your back with legs hip width distance apart, left leg bent with left foot flat on the floor, right leg stretched straight on the floor and arms by your side.

*Steps:*

1.  Pull your navel in engaging the core muscles and raise your right leg up, 2 inches above the mat, as you exhale. Pull your right foot towards you in this position.
2.  Keep breathing and hold this position for 5 counts.
3.  Slowly lower your leg down and come to start position, releasing the imprint, as you inhale.
4.  Repeat this on left side.
5.  Repeat 5 times on each side.

## Back Imprinting with One Knee to Chest

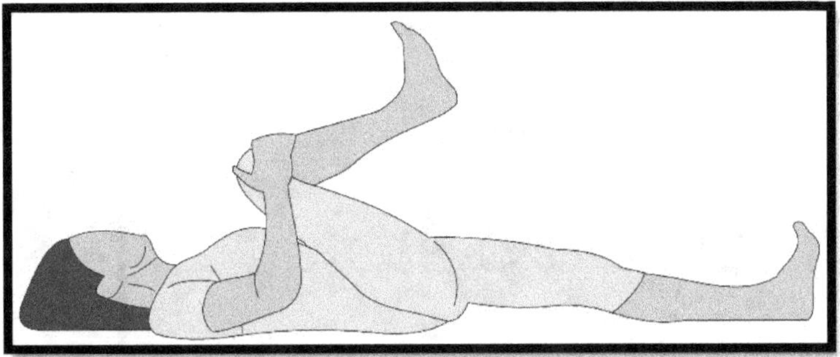

*Effect:* This exercise helps in core strengthening and improves flexion at hip and knee.

*Start Position:* Lie down straight on your back with legs straight on the mat, and feet shoulder width apart.

*Steps:*

1. Do back imprinting and take your right knee towards the chest.
2. Hold your knee there for 5 counts, with your hands around or behind the knee, as you keep on imprinting.
3. Keep on breathing as you hold the above position.
4. Slowly release the position and get your leg back to start position as you inhale.
5. Repeat on the left side.
6. Repeat on each side 5 times.

## Back Imprinting with Both Knees to Chest

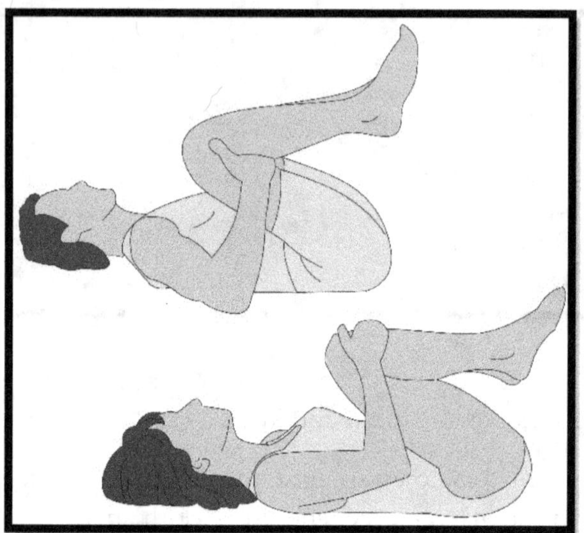

*Effect:* This exercise works on core strengthening and improves flexion at hips and knees.

*Start Position:* Lie down straight on your back with legs bent and feet flat on the mat, hip width distance apart.

*Steps:*

1. Do back imprinting and take your knees towards your chest as you exhale.
2. Hold your knees there for 5 counts, with your hands around or behind the knees, as you continue to imprint the back.
3. Keep breathing as you hold the above position.
4. Slowly release the position and get your knees back to start position as you inhale. Repeat 10 times.

# Back Imprinting with Knees Pressing on the Ball

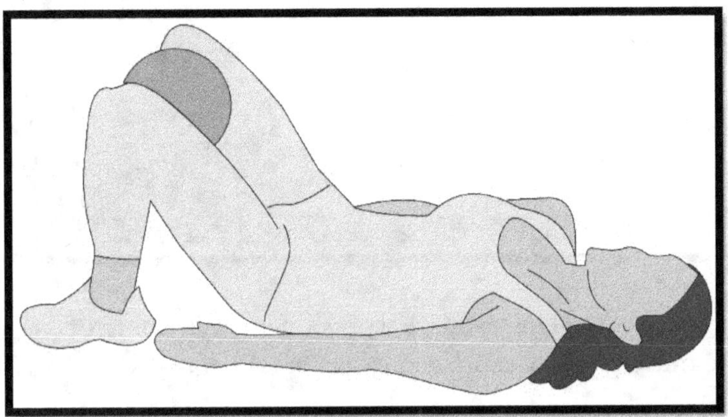

*Effect:* This exercise helps in strengthening of core and adductor muscles.

*Start Position:* Lie down on your back with your legs bent, feet flat on the ground, hip width distance apart and arms by your side. Place a ball (or a fat cushion) between your knees and hold it there.

*Steps:*

1. Do back imprinting as you exhale and press the ball between your knees.
2. Keep breathing and hold this position for 5 counts.
3. Inhale and release the press.
4. Repeat this 10 times.

## Back Imprinting with Heel Slide

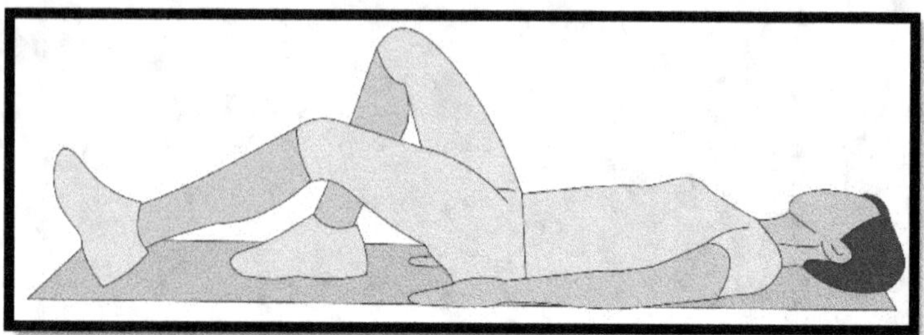

*Effect:*        This exercise works on strengthening of core muscles and flexors and extensors of leg.

*Start Position:*    Lie down on your back with legs bent, shoulder width apart, feet flat on the mat and arms by the side of your body.

*Steps:*

1. Do back imprinting and slide the left foot away from your body in a straight line as you exhale.
2. Inhale and slide the foot back to the start position releasing the imprint.
3. Repeat on the right side.
4. Repeat 5 times on each side.

# Bridging with Arms by Side of Body

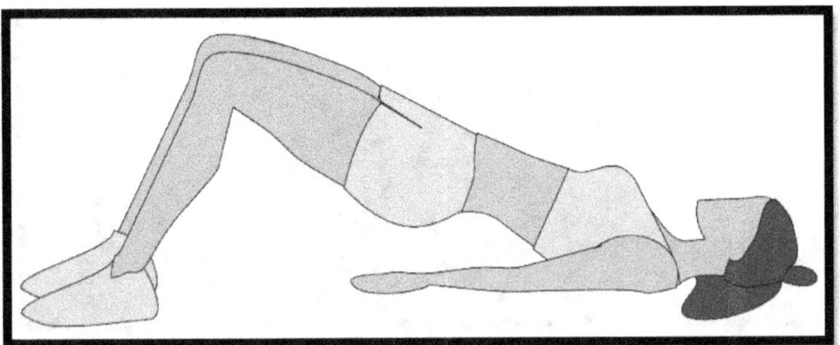

*Effect:*  This is a core strengthening exercise focusing on strengthening of gluteal muscles.

*Start Position:*  Lie down on your back, with legs bent to 90 degrees at hip and knee, feet flat on the mat, shoulder width apart and arms with palms down, by your side.

*Steps:*

1. Exhale, do back imprinting, squeeze your gluteal muscles and raise your hips up, till your knees, hips and shoulder are in one line.
2. Hold this position for 5 counts as you keep shallow breathing.
3. Inhale, release the position and come back to the start position.
4. Repeat this exercise 5 times.

*Fine Tips:*

1. Do not let your knees go apart as you do the bridging.

## Bridging with Arms across the Chest

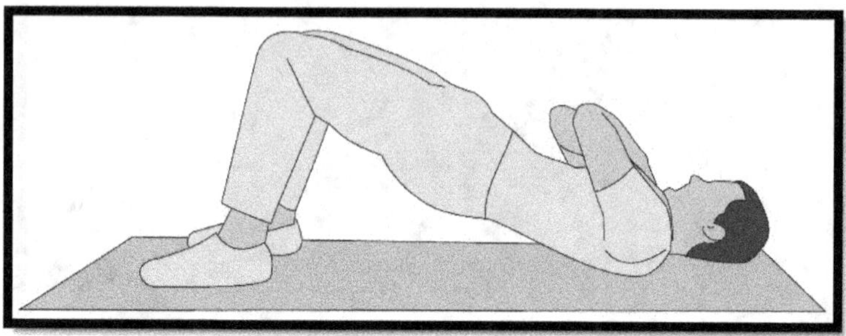

Do bridging (as in earlier exercise, Bridging with Arms by Side of Body) but with arms across your chest.

## Bridging with Single Leg Raise

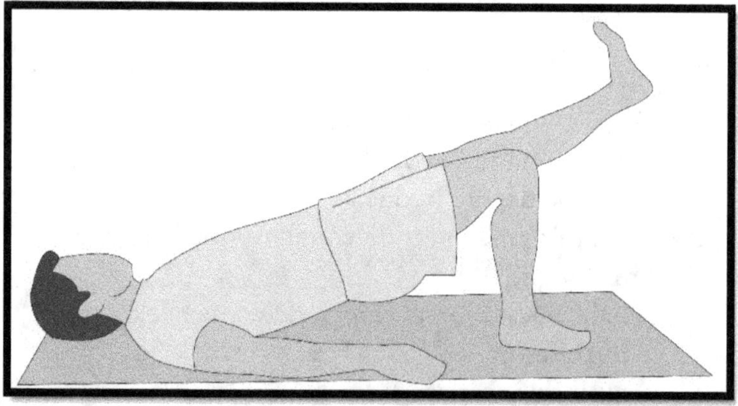

Do bridging (as in earlier exercise, Bridging with Arms by Side of Body) and raise your left leg till it comes in line with right thigh. Release the position and repeat on the right side. Repeat 5 times on each side.

## Bridging with Single Leg Marching

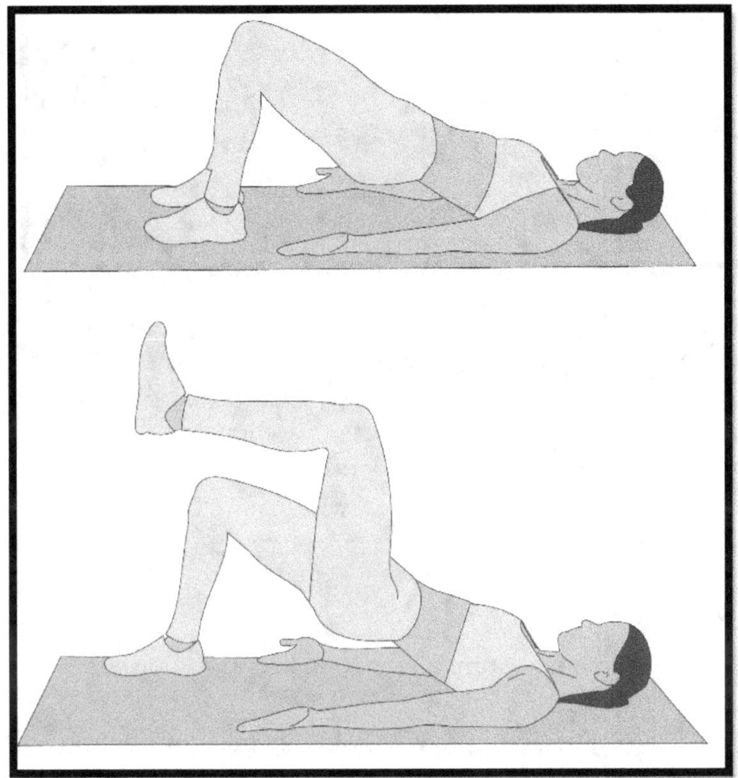

Do bridging (as in earlier exercise, Bridging with Arms by Side of Body). From bridge position start marching by raising right and left leg alternately. Maintain the correct alignment as you march. Repeat 10 times.

## Planks

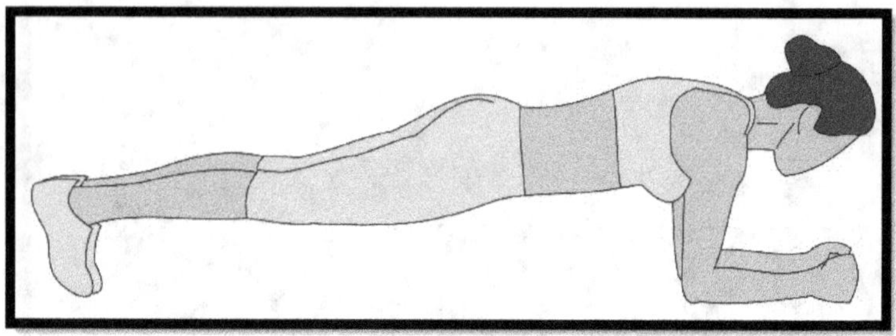

*Effect:* This is a full body strengthening exercise focusing more on core strength.

*Start Position:* Lie down on your abdomen with forearms, elbows on the mat. Raise your body, so that you are resting on your forearms and your toes, with your elbow directly under your shoulders.

*Steps:*

1. Maintain abdominal draw in, keeping your back completely straight.
2. Keep breathing as you hold this position for 15 seconds.
3. Release the position.
4. Repeat it 5 times.
5. Progress in increments of 15 seconds.

## Side Planks

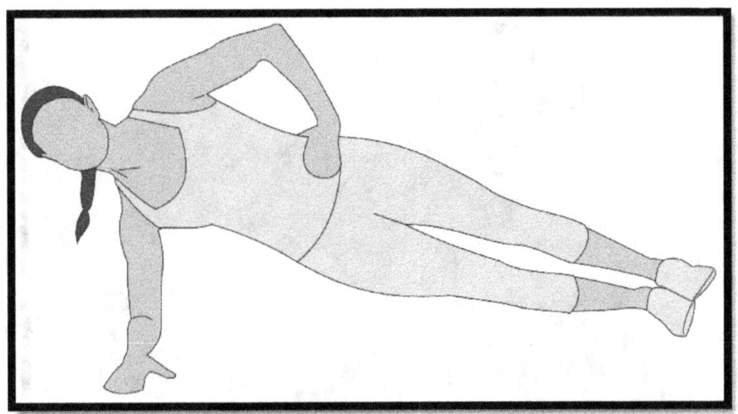

*Effect:*    This is a full body strengthening exercise focusing more on core muscles.

*Start Position:*    Lie down on your side with your elbow underneath you.

*Steps:*

1. Raise yourself on the forearm, resting on the forearm and foot, with your elbow under the shoulder. Your neck, torso, hips and legs should be in one straight line.
2. Hold this position as you keep on breathing for 15 seconds.
3. Return to the start position.
4. Repeat on the other side.
5. Repeat 4-5 times on each side.
6. Progress in increments of 15 seconds.

## Upper Chest Raise on Forearms

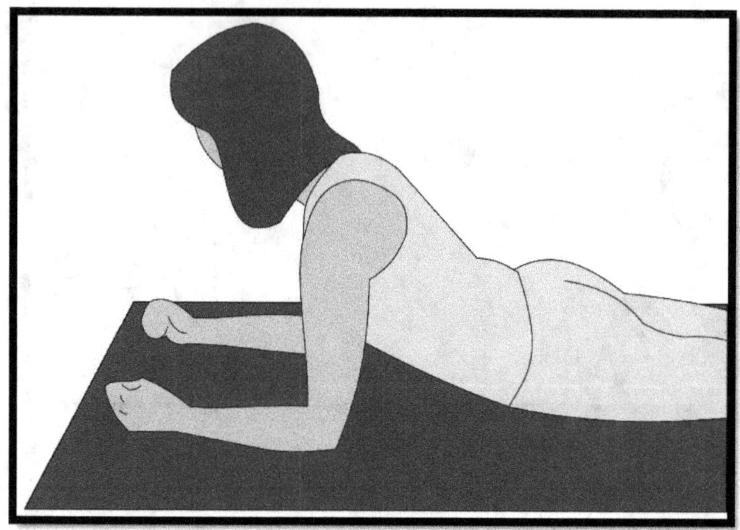

_Effect:_     This exercise helps in stretching of your abdominal muscle and increasing the lumbar lordosis.

_Start Position:_   Lie down on your abdomen with your hands slightly ahead of the shoulders and forearms resting on the mat.

_Steps:_

1.  Inhale and retract your shoulder blades up and in towards the midline of the spine. Push yourself up on the forearm so that your elbows are directly under the shoulders. Your neck and spine should be in one line.
2.  Hold this position for 5 counts.
3.  Return to the start position. Repeat it 5 times.

## Chest Raise till Navel (Cobra Pose)

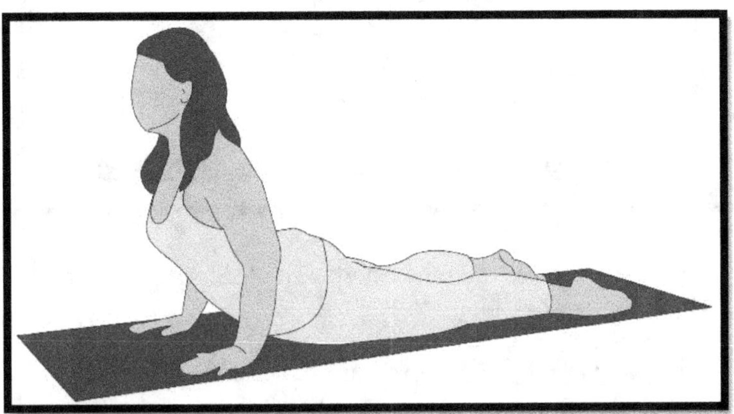

*Effect:* This exercise helps in stretching of your abdominal muscle and increasing the lumbar lordosis.

*Start Position:* Lie down on your abdomen with hands placed under the shoulders.

*Steps:*

1. Push through the hands and raise your chest up with hands remaining under shoulders.
2. Hold this position for 5 counts and return to the start position.
3. Repeat chest raise but this time raise yourself up till naval keeping hands under shoulders.
4. Hold this position for 5 counts and return to the start position.
5. Repeat 5 times.

## Superman Pose

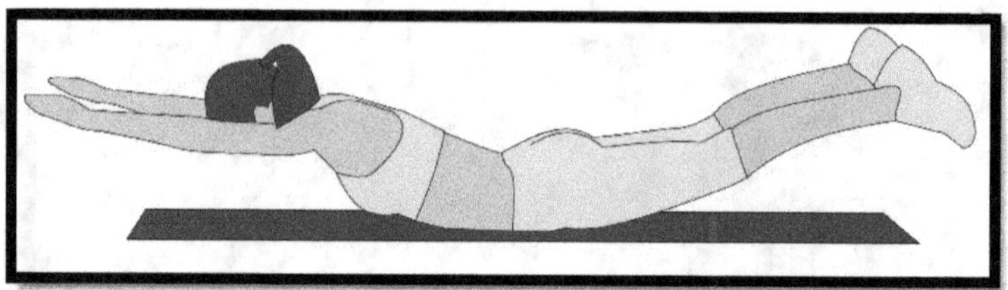

*Effect:*   This exercise works on strengthening of body extensor muscles.

*Start Position:*   Lie down on your abdomen with arms extended ahead. Retract your shoulder blades up and in towards the midline of the spine and draw in the abdominal muscles.

*Steps:*

1. Maintaining the start position, lift up your arms and legs, ensuring your hips stay in contact with the mat.
2. Hold this position for 5 counts as you keep on breathing.
3. Return to the start position.
4. Repeat it 5 times.

## Opposite Arm & Leg Raise in all Fours

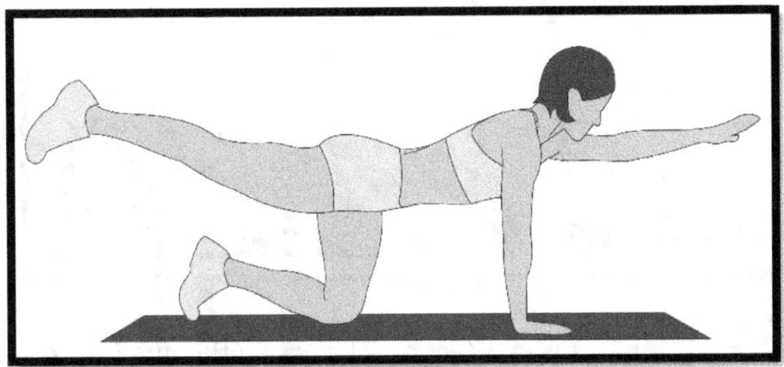

*Effect:* This exercise helps in strengthening of core and extensors of arms and legs.

*Start Position:* Come in all fours position with your hands under the shoulders and knees under the hips. Your neck should be in line with the spine.

*Steps:*

1. Engage your core (draw in your abdominal muscle) and your lower back, hip and hamstring muscles to raise your right leg. Simultaneously raise your left arm.
2. Hold this position for 5 counts.
3. Return to the start position and repeat on the other side.
4. Repeat it 5 times on each side.

## Single Leg Raise in Prone

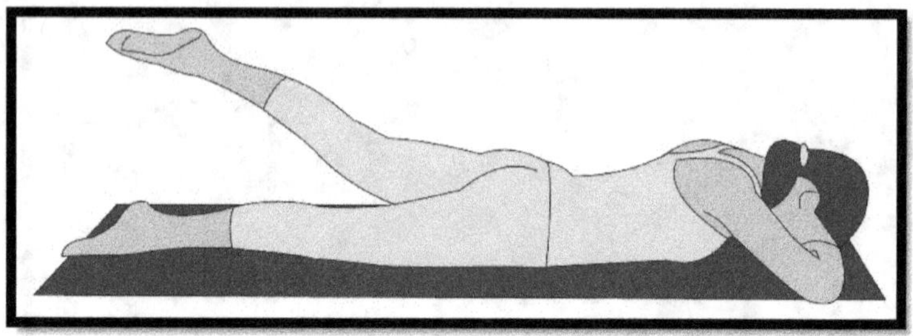

*Effect:*  This exercise helps in strengthening of the extensors of legs especially gluteal muscles.

*Start Position:*  Lie down on your abdomen with your arms bent and your forehead resting on your arms and legs hip width distance apart.

*Steps:*

1.  Squeeze your buttocks and raise left leg straight up.
2.  Hold the position for 5 counts and return to the start position.
3.  Repeat on the right side.
4.  Repeat 5 times on each side.

## Pelvic Tilt on Physio ball

*Effect:*  This is a core strengthening exercise.

*Start Position:*  Sit on the physio ball with your spine tall, knees and hips bent at 90 degrees, legs hip width distance apart, feet flat on the ground and hands on the hips.

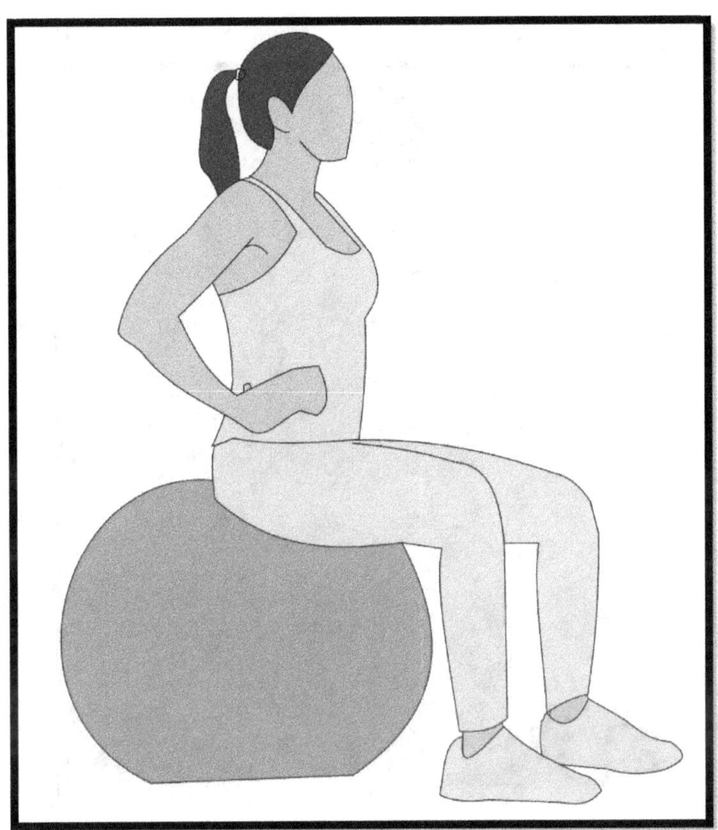

_Steps:_

1. Draw your abdomen in, tighten your gluteal muscles and straighten your lumbar curve as you inhale.
2. Hold this position for 5 counts.
3. Exhale and release the position regaining the lumbar curve.
4. Repeat it 5 times.

## Pelvic Side to Side Shift

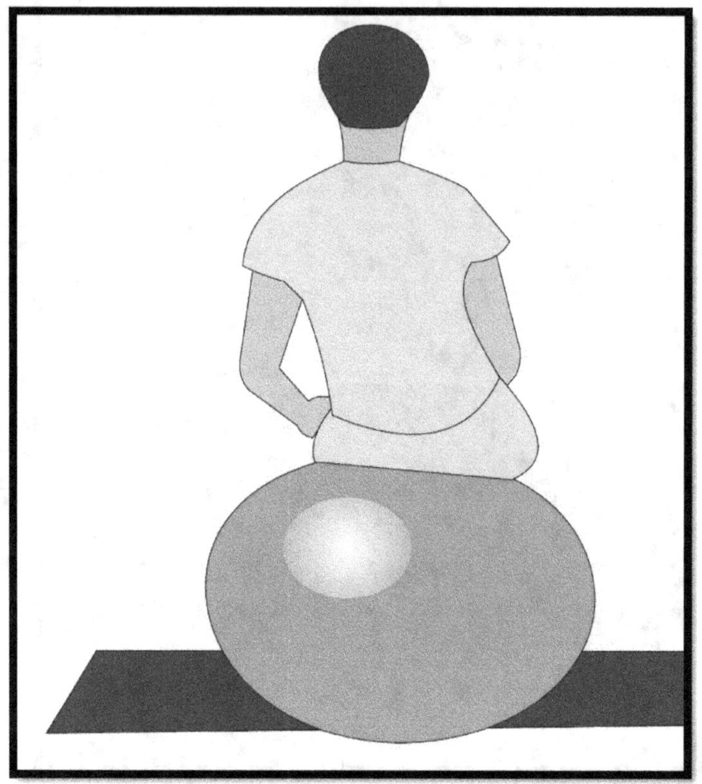

*Effect:*     This is a core strengthening exercise which specifically targets strengthening of trunk side flexors.

*Start Position:*   Sit tall on the physio ball, with knees bent at 90 degrees, feet flat on the ground, hip width apart and hands on the thighs.

*Steps:*

1. Shift your hips to the right so that the physio ball moves with you.
2. Reverse and slide to the opposite side.
3. Repeat this movement 5 times on each side.

*Fine Tips:*

1. Your back should remain tall and shoulders levelled throughout the exercise.


## Pelvic Side to Side Shift with Pelvic Tilt

*Effect:* This is a combination of pelvic tilt and pelvic side to side shifts, making pelvis move in a circle. This works on strengthening of core muscles.

*Start Position:* Sit on the physio ball with knees bent at 90 degrees, feet flat on the ground, shoulder width apart and hands on the hips. Keep your spine tall and shoulders levelled throughout the exercise.

*Steps:*

1. Begin by drawing your abdomen in, straightening your lumbar curve.
2. Then slide your hips to the right side.
3. Next, move your hips forward.
4. Finally move your hips to the left side.
5. Repeat this sequence 10 times in one direction and then 10 times in opposite direction.

## Pelvic Tilt with Leg Marching

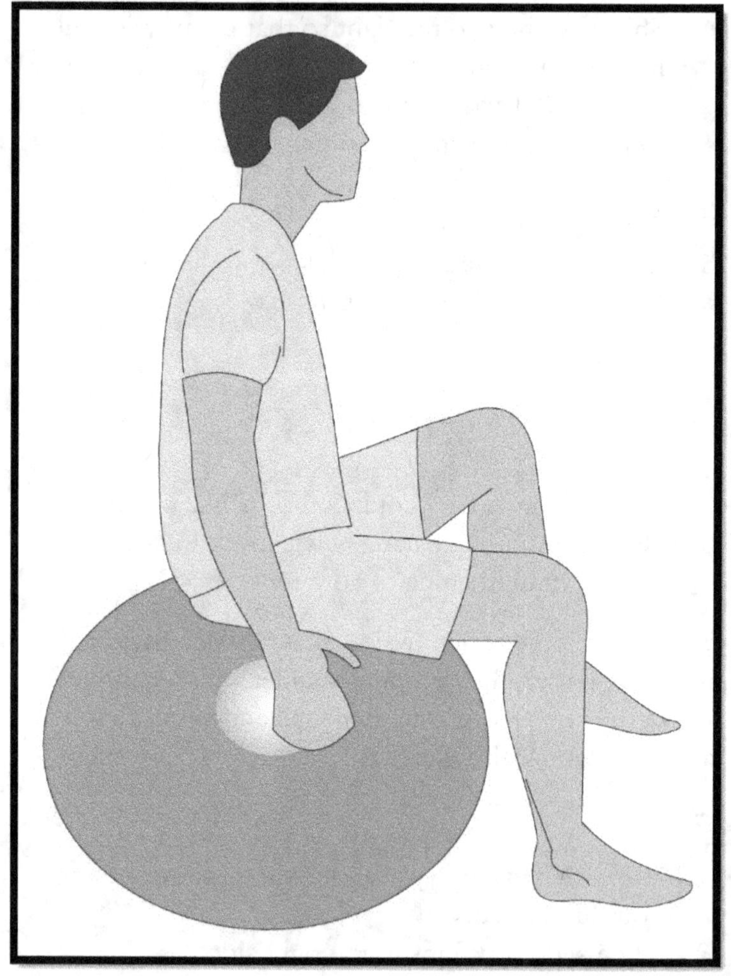

*Effect:*  This exercise works on strengthening of core muscles with emphasis on hip flexors.

*Start Position:*  Sit tall on the physio ball with knees bent at 90 degrees, feet flat on the ground, hip width distance apart, and arms by the side of the body with hands rested on the ball.

*Steps:*

1. Draw your abdomen in and maintain this throughout the exercise.
2. Keeping your hips levelled focus on the left knee and hip, raising the left knee up.
3. Get it down to the start position and repeat on the right side.
4. Repeat it 15-20 times.

## Pelvic Tilt with Leg Raise on Physio Ball

*Effect:*  This is a core muscles strengthening exercise with emphasis on knee extensors.

*Start Position:*  Sit tall on the physio ball, with knees bent at 90 degrees and feet flat on the ground hip width distance apart.

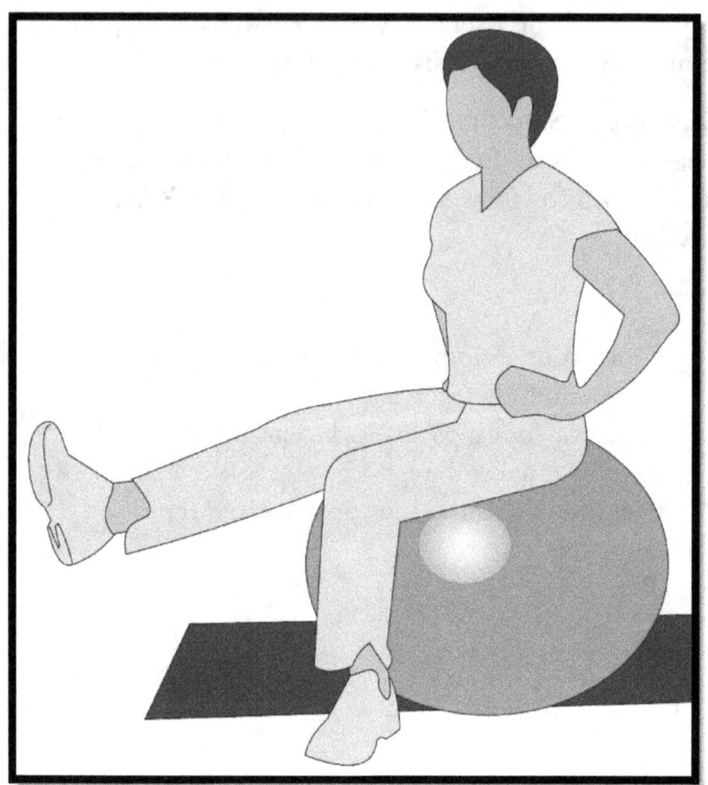

<u>*Steps:*</u>

1.  Tuck your abdomen in and maintain this position as you raise your lower leg up to thigh level, pulling the foot towards you.
2.  Hold this position for 5 counts and slowly lower the leg down to the start position.
3.  Repeat it on the other side.
4.  Repeat it 5 times on each side.

# MEDIUM STRENGTHENING EXERCISES FOR BACK

Back Imprinting with Alternate Arm & Leg Stretch

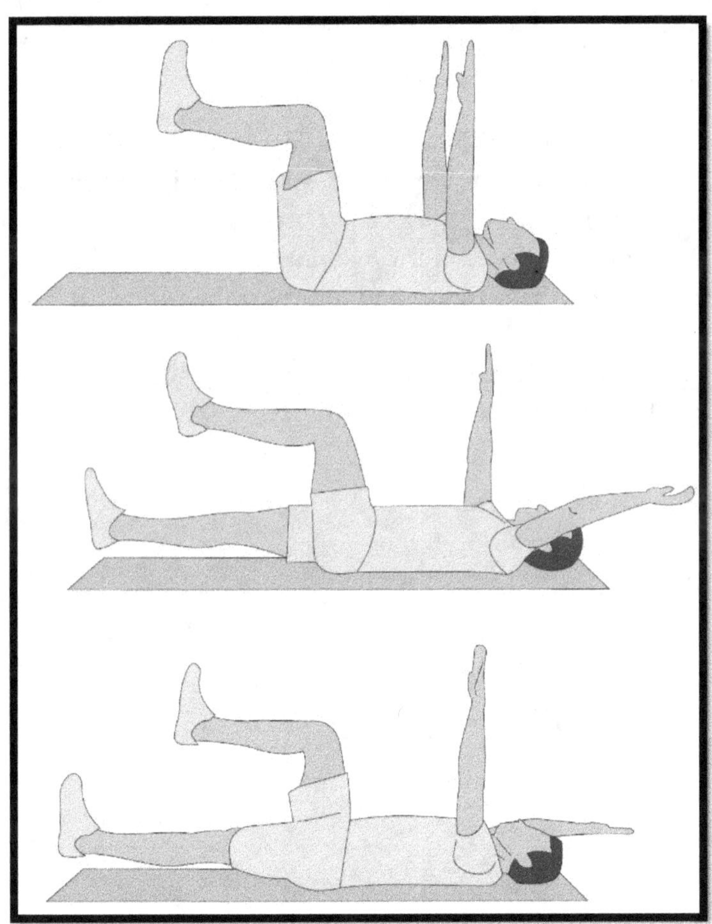

*Effect:*		This is a core strengthening exercise which also helps to strengthen your arms and legs flexors and extensors.

*Start Position:*	Lie down on your back with arms perpendicular to the body and hips and knees bent at 90 degrees, and feet hip width distance apart.

*Steps:*

1. Draw your abdomen in and maintain it as you stretch your left arm overhead and straighten your right leg.
2. Hold this position for 5 counts.
3. Release the position and return to the start position.
4. Repeat it on the other side.
5. Repeat this movement 10 times.

## Back Imprinting with Feet on the Ball

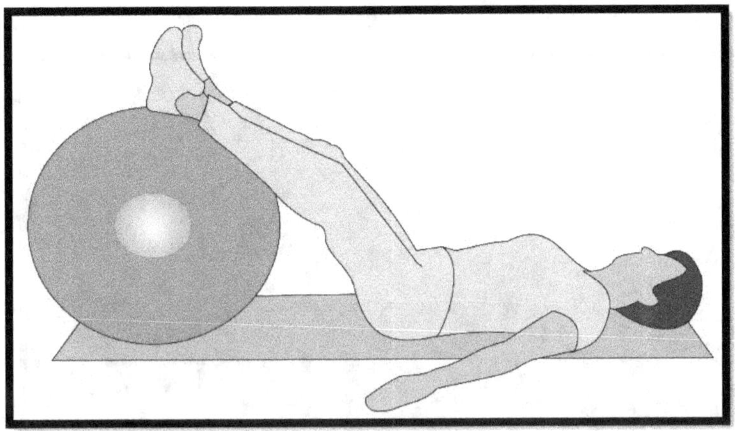

*Effect:*  This exercise works on core strengthening with legs in flexed position.

*Start Position:*  Lie down on the mat with hips and knees bent at 45 degrees and feet placed on the physio ball.

*Steps:*

1. Draw your abdomen in and imprint your back on the mat, as you exhale, in this position.
2. Hold for 5 counts.
3. Slowly release the imprint as you inhale and return to the start position.
4. Repeat 5 times.

## Back Imprinting with Arms and Legs raise and Partial Sit-up

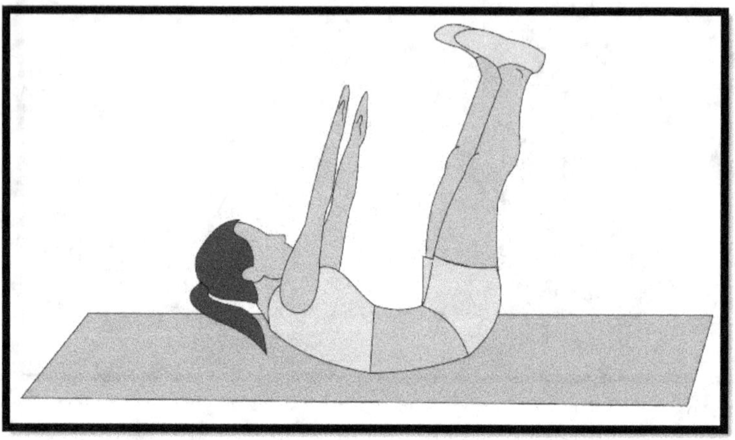

*Effect:*        This is a core strengthening exercise focusing on toning of upper and lower abdominal muscles.

*Start Position:*    Do back imprinting in supine position, with knees and hips bent at 90 degrees and knees hip width distance apart.

*Steps:*

1.  Raise the shoulder and head off the floor, just to the point where shoulder blades are barely touching the floor as if trying to grab a trapeze. Straighten your legs simultaneously.
2.  Hold the above position for 1-2 seconds.
3.  Return to the start position as you inhale. Repeat the same sequence 10-15 times.

# Rolling To & Fro

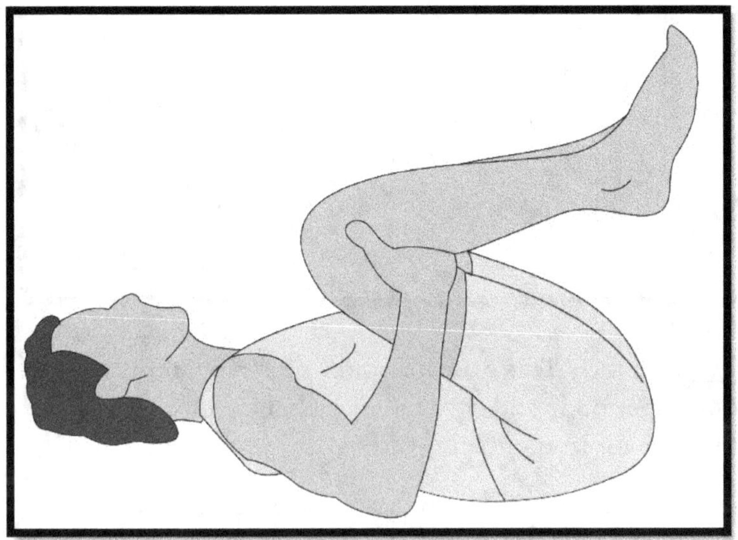

*Effect:* This is a core strengthening exercise which also helps in stretching of back muscles and lower limb extensors.

*Start Position:* Sit in a tucked position and draw your abdomen in, holding back side of your thigh.

*Steps:*

1. Roll back on your shoulder blades, then roll forward to the start position.
2. Repeat this movement 20 times.

## Plank with Single Leg Raise

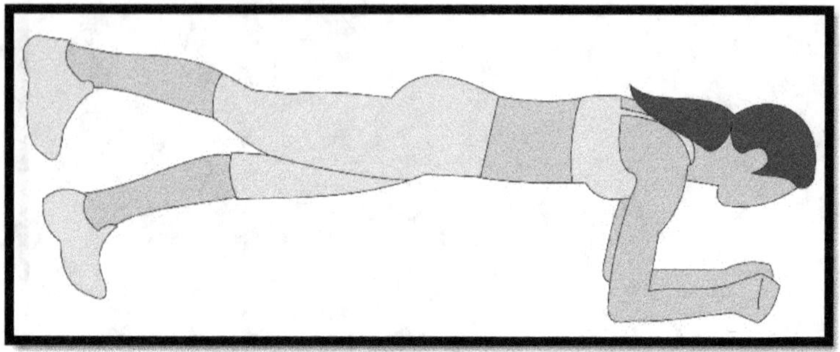

*Effect:*        This exercise works on strengthening of your upper body and core muscles along with extra emphasis on strengthening of hip extensors.

*Start Position:*    Lie down on your abdomen with your elbows underneath your shoulders.

*Steps:*

1. Push your body up on the forearms as you draw in the abdomen. Your body should be resting on your forearms and toes, with your elbows directly under the shoulders and neck, back and hips in one line.
2. Maintain the above position and raise your right leg straight up.
3. Hold for 5 counts.
4. Lower the leg to start position.
5. Raise the left leg up.
6. Repeat 5 times on each side.

## Side Plank with One Leg Abduction

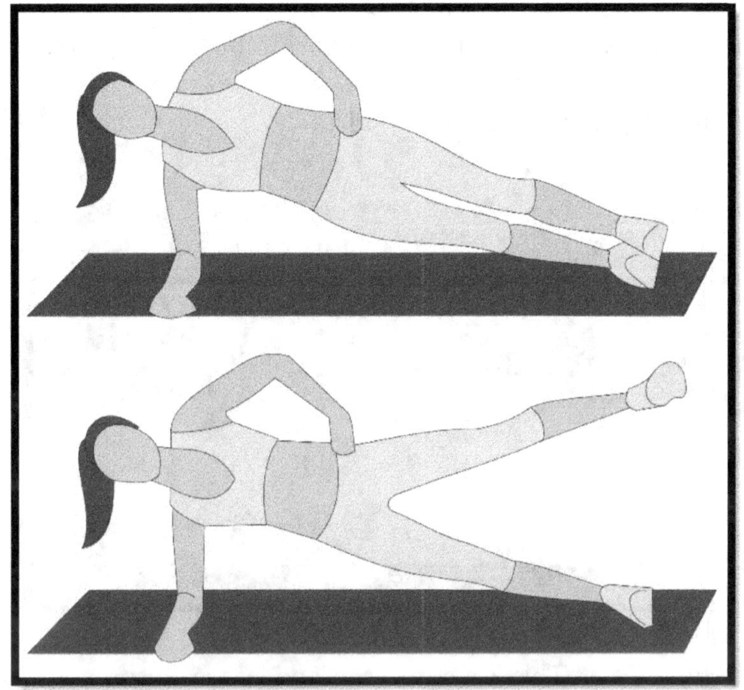

*Effect:*      This exercise helps in strengthening of your core muscles and abductors (side movement muscles) of your arms and legs.

*Start Position:*   Lie down on your right side with your elbow underneath you.

*Steps:*

1. Push yourself up so that your body is resting on the right forearm (elbow under the shoulder) and the right foot.

2. Hold this position as you raise your left leg up.
3. Hold this position for 5 counts.
4. Release the position and come to the start position.
5. Repeat it 5 times.
6. Repeat it on the other side.

## Diagonal Arm / Leg Extension with Weight Cuffs

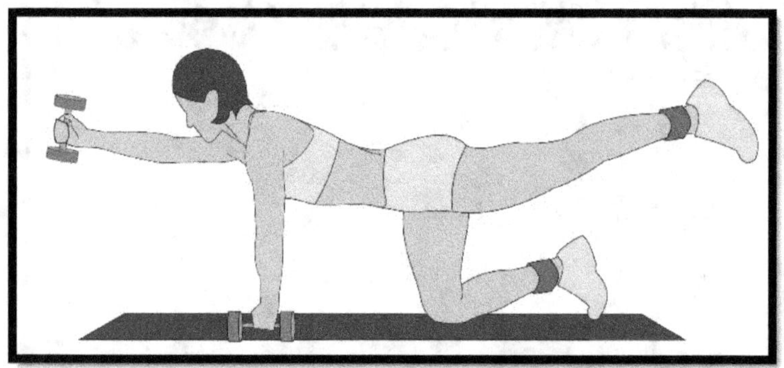

*Effect:* This is a core, arms and legs extensors strengthening exercise.

*Start Position:* Tie weight cuffs around your ankles and hold dumbbells in your hands. Get into all fours position with hands under the shoulders and knees under the hips. Tuck in your abdomen and maintain this position.

*Steps:*

1. Contract your low back, hip and hamstring muscles and lift a leg with weight cuff up and also raise the diagonally opposite arm with dumbbell maintaining the all fours position.

2.  Your raised leg, arm and body are in one plane.
    Hold this position for 5 counts.
3.  Release the position returning to the start position.
4.  Repeat it 10 times on each side.

*Fine Tips:*

1.  Balancing yourself on the dumbbell may be
    difficult, especially with one arm and leg raised.
    You can also do this exercise with weight cuffs on
    wrists.

## Bridging with Legs on Physio Ball

*Effect:*　　　　This is a core strengthening exercise that
focuses on strengthening of gluteal and low back extensor
muscles.

*Start Position:*　Lie down on your back with your feet
resting on the physio ball and arms by the side of your
body with palms down.

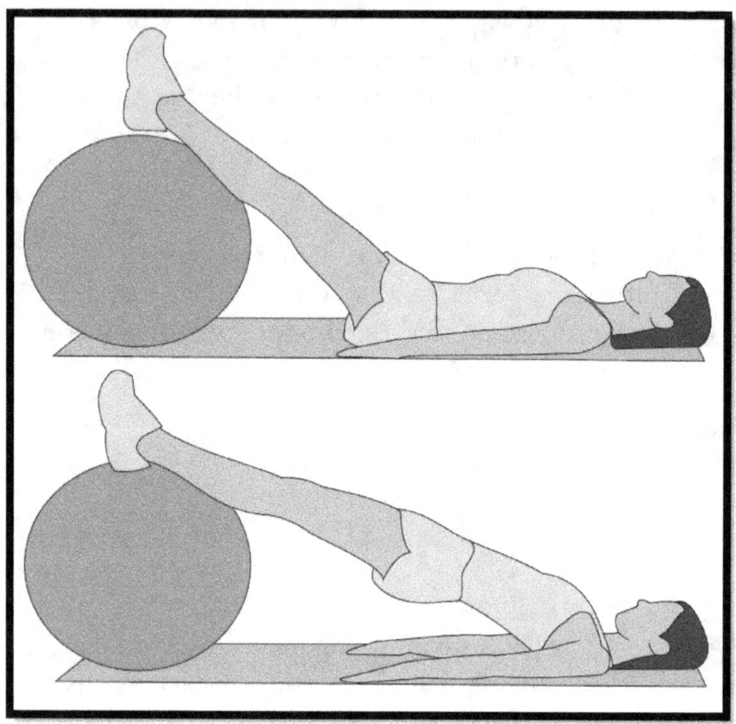

<u>*Steps:*</u>

1. Tuck in your abdomen and maintain this position. Contract your gluteal muscles and raise your hips up, getting your thighs in line with the trunk.
2. Hold this position for 5 counts.
3. Slowly release the position, lowering to the start position.
4. Repeat it 5-10 times.

## Superman Exercise with both Arms & Legs Raise

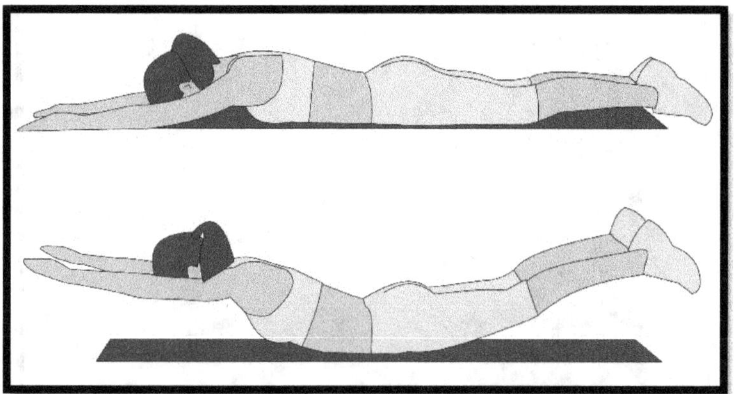

*Effect:* This is a core strengthening exercise which focuses on strengthening of upper back and leg extensor muscles.

*Start Position:* Lie down on your abdomen and stretch your arms overhead.

*Steps:*

1. Contract your lower back, gluteal and hamstring muscles and raise your legs straight up. Raise your chest and arms off the mat.
2. Hold this position for 5 counts.
3. Return to the start position.
4. Repeat it 5 times.

## Abdominal Crunch on Physio Ball

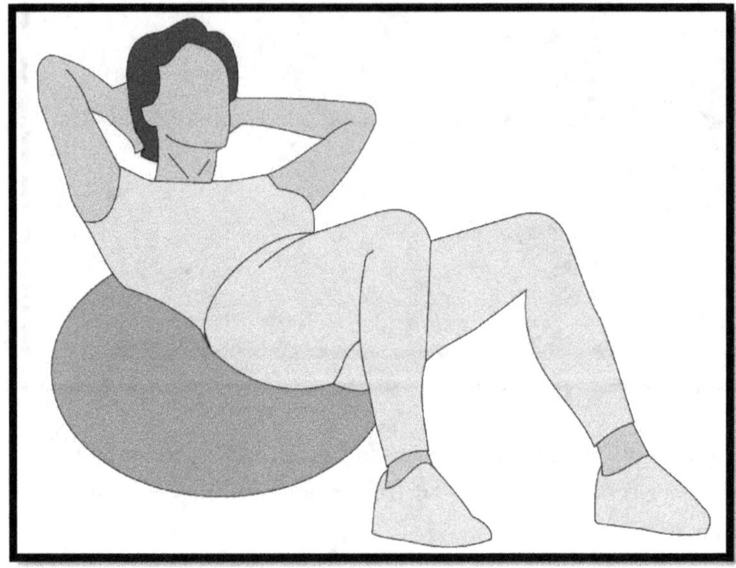

*Effect:* This is a core strengthening exercise that focuses on strengthening of upper abdominal muscles.

*Start Position:* Begin with lying on the physio ball with your hips just off the physio ball. Keep your feet shoulder width apart and place your hands behind your head.

*Steps:*

1. Tuck in your abdomen and maintain. Crunch forward and lift your shoulder blades off the ball.
2. Hold this position at top for 1-2 seconds.
3. Slowly lower back down to the start position.
4. Repeat it 10 times.

## Side Abdominal Crunches

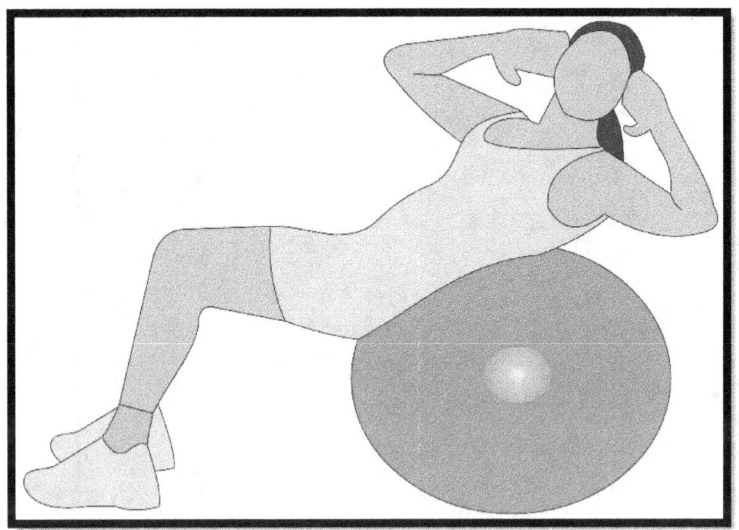

*Effect:* This is a core strengthening exercise that focuses on strengthening of abdominal oblique muscles.

*Start Position:* Begin with your back on the physio ball, hips just off the ball, thighs parallel to the ground and feet flat on the ground shoulder width apart.

*Steps:*

1. Tuck in your abdomen and maintain this position. Get your hands behind the head, crunch forward and lift your shoulder blades off the ball. As you get halfway twist your body to a side.
2. Maintain it at top position for 1-2 seconds.
3. Slowly lower back to the start position.
4. Repeat it 5 times on each side.

## Bridging with Head on Physio Ball

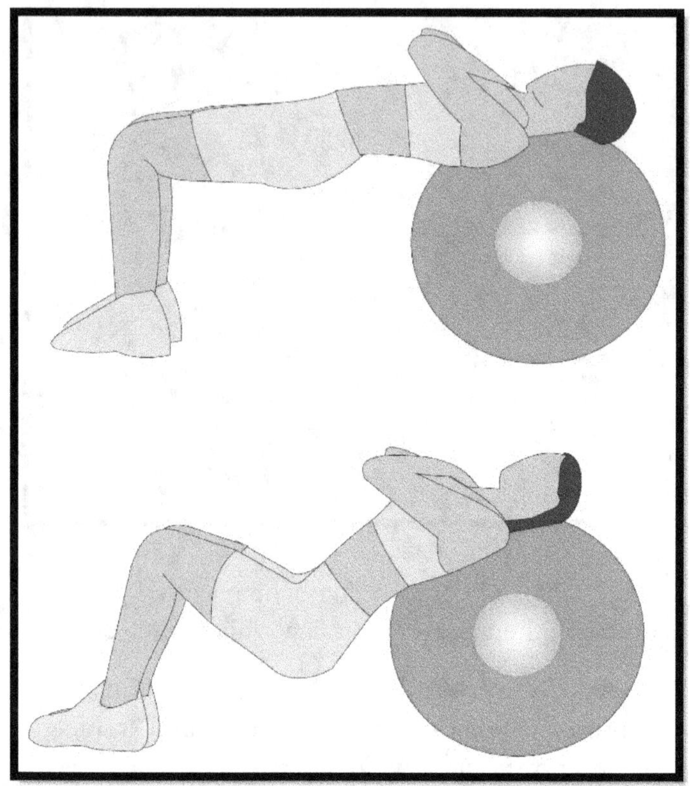

*Effect:*	This is a core strengthening exercise with focus on gluteal and lower back muscle strengthening.

*Start Position:*	Align your shoulder blades on the physio ball with arms across the chest, thighs and hips off the ball and feet shoulder width apart.

*Steps:*

1. Contract your gluteal and hamstring muscles and tuck in your abdomen, getting trunk, hips, thighs and knees in one line.
2. Hold this position for 5 counts.
3. Slowly reverse the movement and return to the start position.
4. Repeat the movement 10 times.

## Pelvic Tilt with Single Leg Raise

*Effect:* This exercise works on strengthening of core muscles with emphasis on knee extensors.

*Start Position:* Sit tall on the physio ball, with knees bent at 90 degrees, feet flat on the ground, hip width distance apart and hands on the hips.

*Steps:*

1. Draw in your abdomen, raise your arm up, and join your hands in the Indian greeting (*Namastey*). Raise right leg straight up, straightening at knee and pull foot and toes towards you as your leg comes in horizontal position.
2. Hold this position for 5 counts and release, returning to the start position.

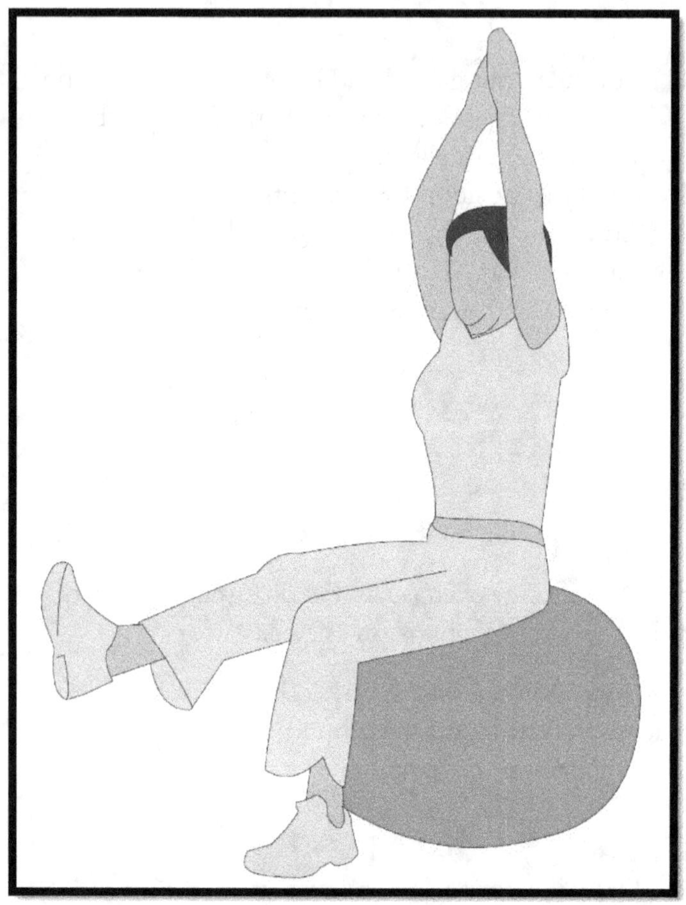

3.  Repeat on the left side.
4.  Repeat 5 times on each side.

# ADVANCED STRENGTHENING EXERCISES

## Plank Walk

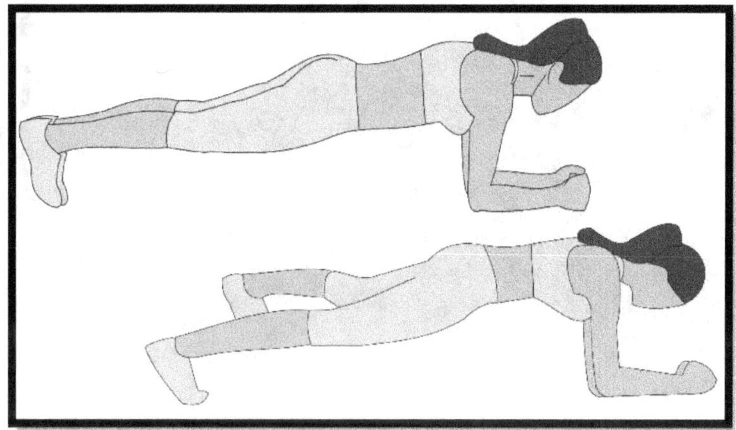

*Effect:*  This is a dynamic core and upper body strengthening exercise.

*Start Position:*  Begin by coming in plank position with body resting on forearms (elbows under the shoulders) and toes.

*Steps:*

1. Tuck your abdomen in, maintaining neck, spine and hips in one line.
2. Step to left side with left leg (left toes), followed by right Leg (right toes) then left arm/hand followed by right arm and hand.
3. Take 4-5 side steps in one direction and then repeat the whole sequence in other direction taking 4-5 steps.

## Side Plank with Leg Flexion & Extension

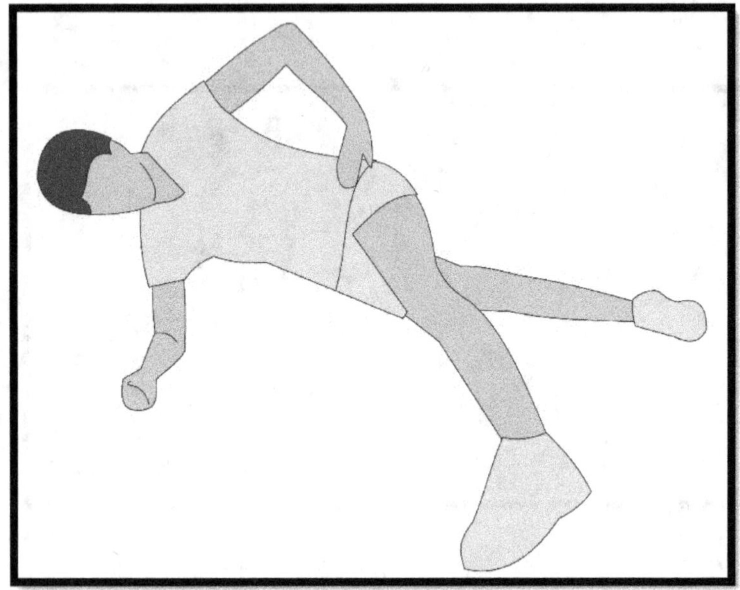

*Effect:* This is a core strengthening exercise with focus on strengthening of leg flexor and extensor muscles.

*Start Position:* Begin by coming in side plank position, with your body resting on forearm underneath your body and side of the foot.

*Steps:*

1. Maintain the start position and lift your top leg. Kick the leg forward and backward.
2. Repeat this movement 5-10 times.
3. Switch the side and repeat on the other side.

## Seated Trunk Twists with Medicine Ball

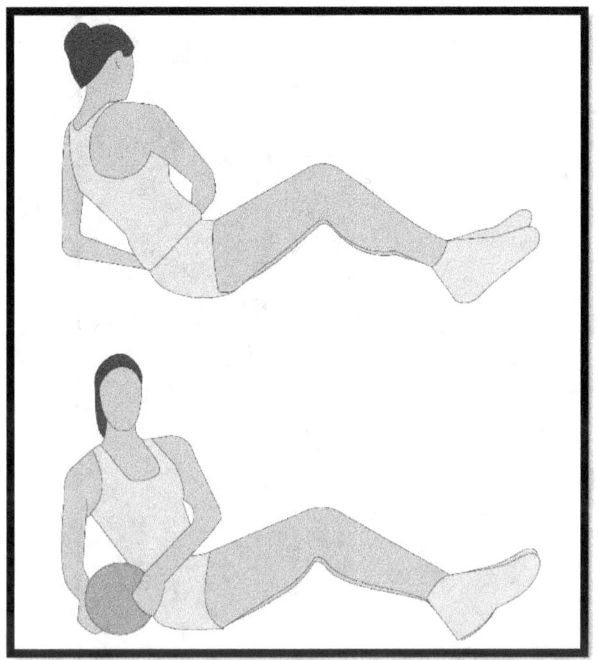

*Effect:* This is a core strengthening exercise targeting the abdominal oblique muscles.

*Start Position:* Sit on the mat engaging your core, hips and knees slightly flexed, holding the medicine ball in your hands.

*Steps:*

1. Turn to the left side and right side with the ball, keeping the core engaged. The twist should begin from abdomen, then chest and finally neck.
2. Repeat it 15-20 times.

## Seated Trunk Twists with Med Ball on Physio Ball

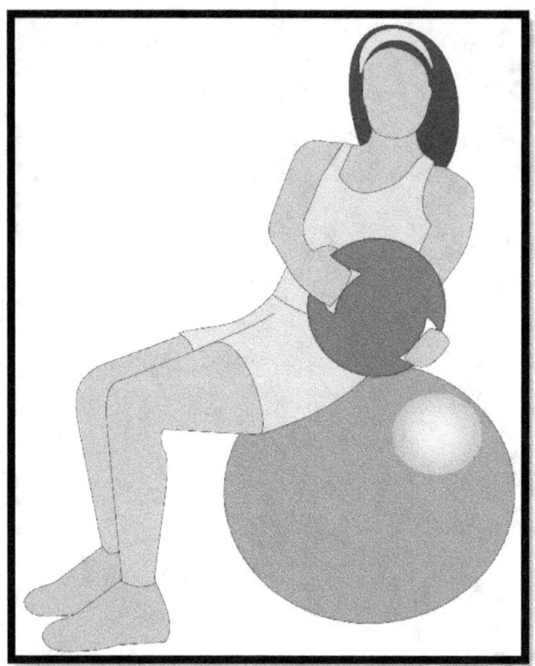

_Effect:_        This is a core strengthening exercise focusing on strengthening of abdominal oblique muscles.

_Start Position:_   Sit tall on the physio ball with the core engaged, feet hip width distance apart and planted on the ground. Hold a medicine ball in front of you.

_Steps:_

1.  Draw your abdomen in and turn to the right side and then to the left. Turn in the sequence of abdomen, chest and neck.
2.  Repeat this movement 15-20 times.

# Bridging with Single Leg Raise from Physio Ball

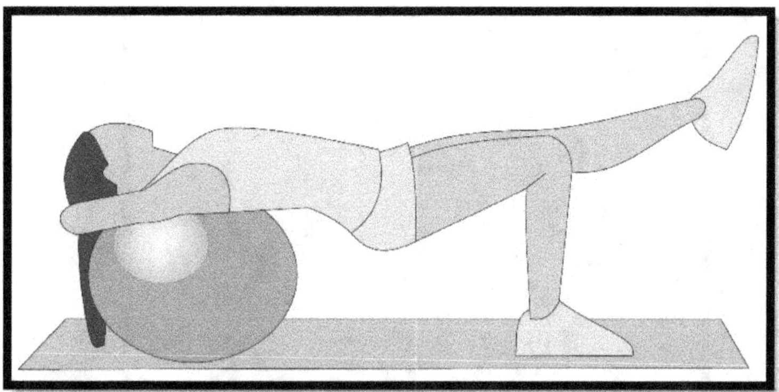

*Effect:* This is a core strengthening exercise targeting hip extensor muscle activation and promoting trunk stability.

*Start Position:* Place your shoulder blades on physio ball with hands behind head and hips just off the physio ball. Maintain the thighs and hips parallel to the floor by contracting lower back, gluteal and hamstring muscles.

*Steps:*

1. Raise your left foot off the ground, extending the leg as you keep your hips levelled.
2. Hold the leg here for 5 counts.
3. Return to the start position.
4. Repeat it on the other side.
5. Repeat 5 times on each side.

## Rolling Push-ups with Medicine Ball

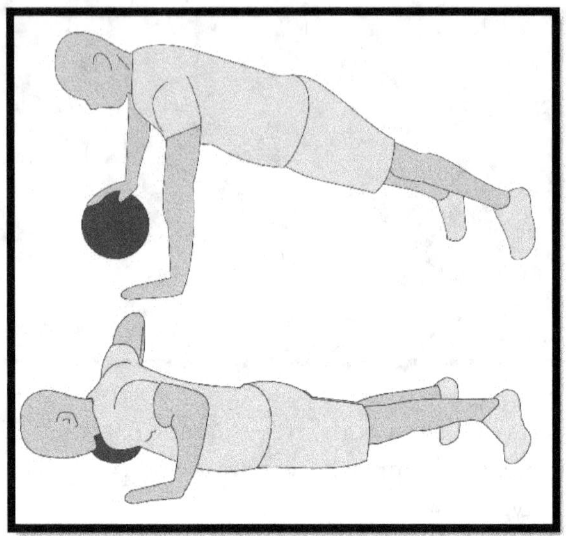

*Effect:*        This exercise helps in strengthening of chest, arm, shoulders and core muscles.

*Start Position:*   Come in a high plank position with your hands under the shoulders and elbows straight. Your body is resting on the hands and toes in this position with your abdomen tucked in throughout the exercise.

*Steps:*

1. Place a medicine ball under one hand in this position.
2. Lower your chest towards the floor to do push up.
3. Return to high plank and roll the ball to the other hand.
4. Repeat this 10 times.

## Weighted Superman with Medicine Ball

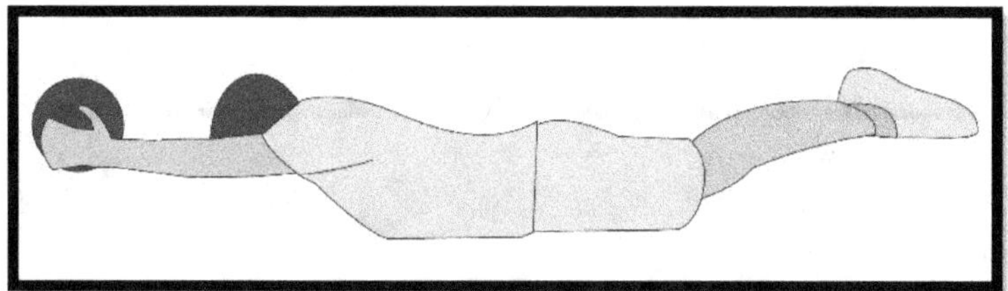

*Effect:*   This exercise helps in strengthening of back extensor and core muscles.

*Start Position:*   Lie down straight on your abdomen with your arms and legs extended and abdomen tucked in throughout the exercise.

*Steps:*

1. Hold a medicine ball in your hands and raise your legs and arms up from the floor engaging your upper back and lower back, gluteal and hamstring muscles.
2. Return to the start position.
3. Repeat it 10 times

## Medicine Ball Fly on Physio Ball

*Effect:*   This is a core strengthening exercise promoting trunk stability and activation of hip extensor muscles with arms weighted abduction.

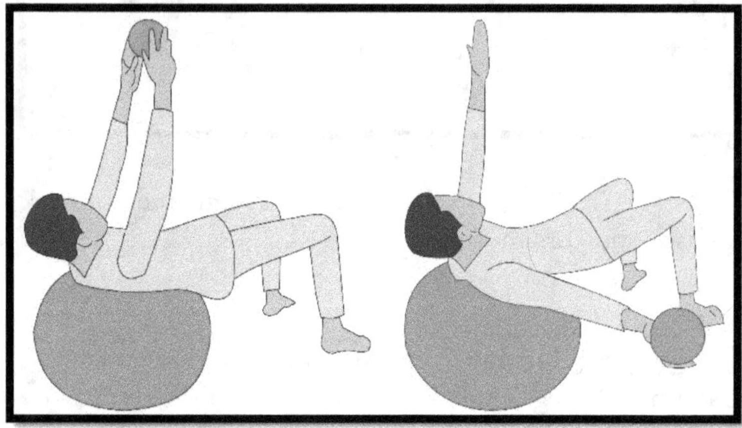

*Start Position:*    Place your shoulder blades on physio ball with arms raised towards the ceiling at 90 degrees to the body, holding the medicine ball in the hands, and hips just off the physio ball. Maintain the thighs and hips parallel to the floor by contracting lower back, gluteal and hamstring muscles.

*Steps:*

1. Grab the medicine ball in right hand and move it sideways to the shoulder level, keeping arms straight at elbow.
2. Slowly bring it back to the start position.
3. Repeat it on the left side.
4. Do 10 repetitions with each hand.

# CHAPTER 7

## Stretching Exercises for Back

Stretching exercises of muscles in lower back, buttocks, hips and legs help to keep them mobile and align the pelvis thus preventing low back pain. Almost everyone can get benefited by these exercises. Stretches reduce the risk of disability caused by back pain as most of them can be done during back pain also.

While stretching, follow the following instructions:

- Hold each stretch for 20-30 seconds to adequately elongate the tight muscle.
- Stretch should be done in the pain free limits. Don't push your body into complex positions for the same.
- Get into the stretch and come out of it slowly. Jerky or fast movements can strain the involved muscles and thus increase spasm.
- As you hold the stretch, breathe into the tight muscles and relax them.
- Repeat each stretch between 2-5 times to attain desired effect.
- If you feel any increase in pain or discomfort with the stretch, stop performing it immediately and consult your doctor or therapist before starting the exercise routine.

- Wear comfortable clothes and lie down on flat large surface to get freedom of movement while stretching.
- Stretching gives best result after myofascial release of the particular muscle or engaging the muscle in aerobic or strengthening exercises.
- Chronic pain (that last for more than 3 months) may need weeks or months of regular stretching to reduce pain.

## Lower Back Twist

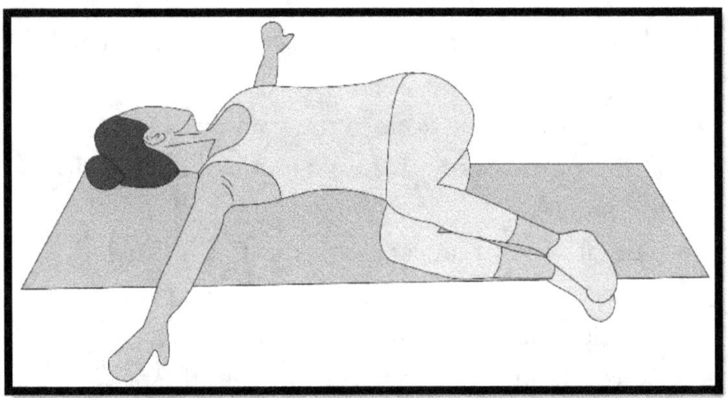

*Effect:* This twist helps to stretch the lower back and gluteal muscles which become tight in low back ache, further increasing the pain.

*Start Position:* Start by lying straight on the ground with knees bent and feet flat on the ground, hip width distance apart. Stretch your arms to the side at shoulder level, making a 'T' with your body.

<u>*Steps:*</u>

1.  Drop your knees to right side slowly as you exhale and turn your face to the left side.
2.  Keep your shoulders on the ground as you do this movement
3.  Hold this position for 30 seconds. Keep breathing into the contracted back and gluteal muscles, thereby relaxing them.
4.  Inhale and get the legs back to start position.
5.  Repeat this on the other side.

<u>*Fine Tips:*</u>

1.  If the stretch is too much, keep a pillow or stack of blankets under your knees when you turn to each side.

## Child's Pose

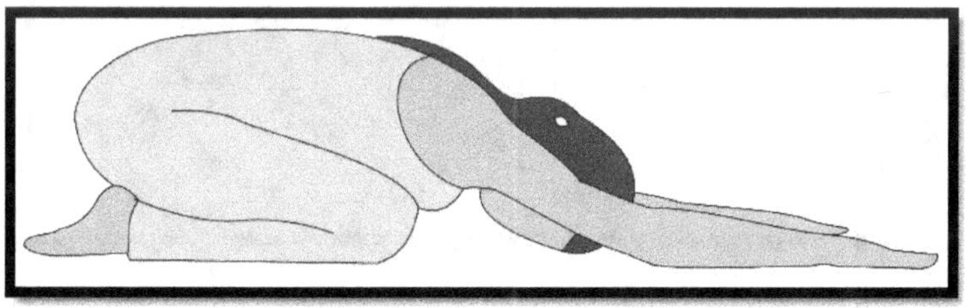

<u>*Effect:*</u>    This posture helps to stretch the muscles of low back which are most likely to be contracted in low back pain.

*Start Position:*    Start by coming in all fours position (with hands and feet on the floor, hands under the shoulders and knees under the hips).

*Steps:*

1.  Stretch your arms in front (sliding your hands on the floor). Slowly sit back on your heels and drop your head and chest downwards as you extend your arms further.
2.  Breathe into the tight back muscles in this position and let the contracted muscles relax.
3.  Hold this position for 20-30 seconds.

## Pelvic Tilt

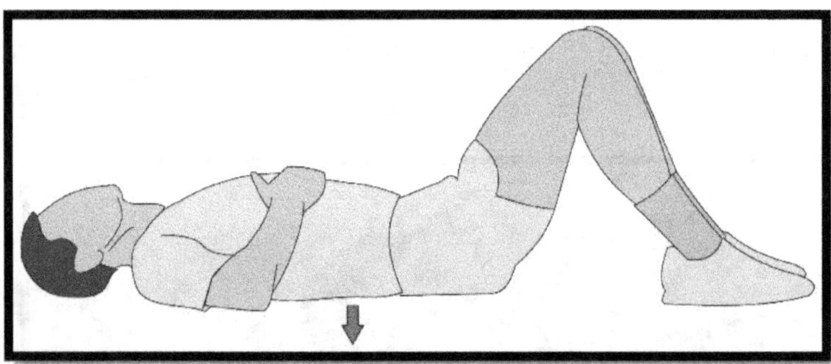

*Effect:*                 When you are having back pain you may feel the entire back is immovable. Pelvic tilt exercise helps to bring back the movement to this area gently. This exercise activates the core muscles taking off the extra work which is to be done by back muscle in supporting the spine.

*Start Position:*    Begin by lying down on the mat with knees bent and feet flat on the mat. Try to relax your back keeping it in neutral position (i.e. if you place the hand under your back you should feel a slight curve).

*Steps:*

1. Take your naval in (engage your core) and flatten your back on the mat (imprint your back) as you exhale.
2. Hold the imprint for 5 counts as you continue with shallow breathing.
3. Inhale and release the imprint slowly as you inhale.
4. Repeat this 10 times.

## Cat & Camel Pose

*Effect:*        This is the dynamic movement of the back that moves the back in two directions. It helps to soothe the soreness in the back, lengthens the contracted muscles and increases the spine mobility.

*Start Position:*    Start by coming on all fours (hands and knees on floor, hands under the shoulder and knees under the hips). Your spine should be parallel to floor in this position.

*Steps:*

1. Tighten the abdominal muscles and arch your spine upwards towards the ceiling as you exhale.

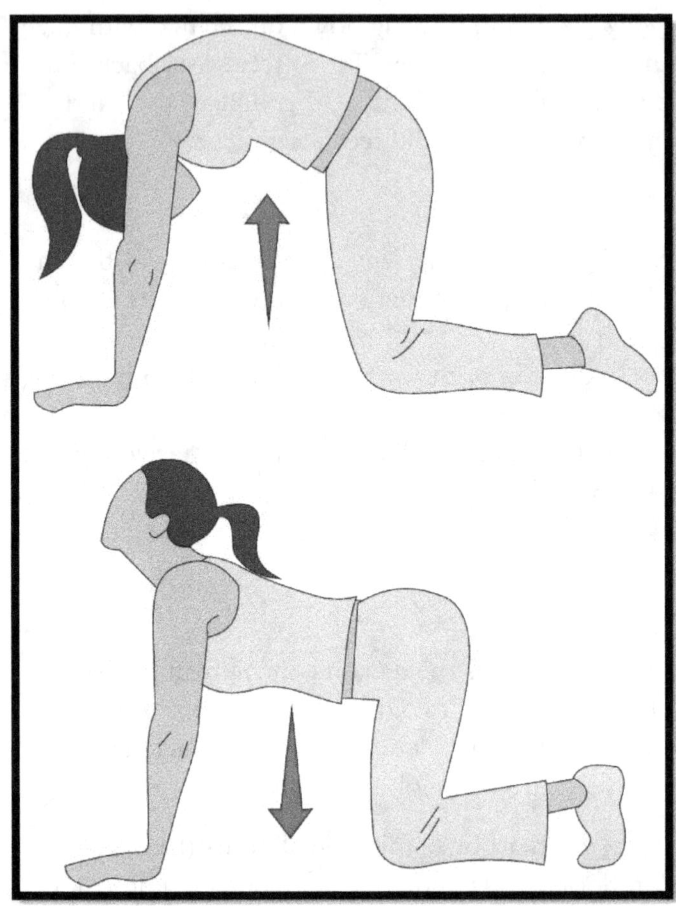

2. Hold this position for 5 counts and then relax your back.
3. Next let your abdomen fall towards the floor, stretching your back downwards into a swayback position, bringing your shoulders together. Inhale.
4. Hold this position chop 5 counts and then relax.
5. Repeat above sequence for 20 seconds.

## Piriformis Figure of Four Stretch

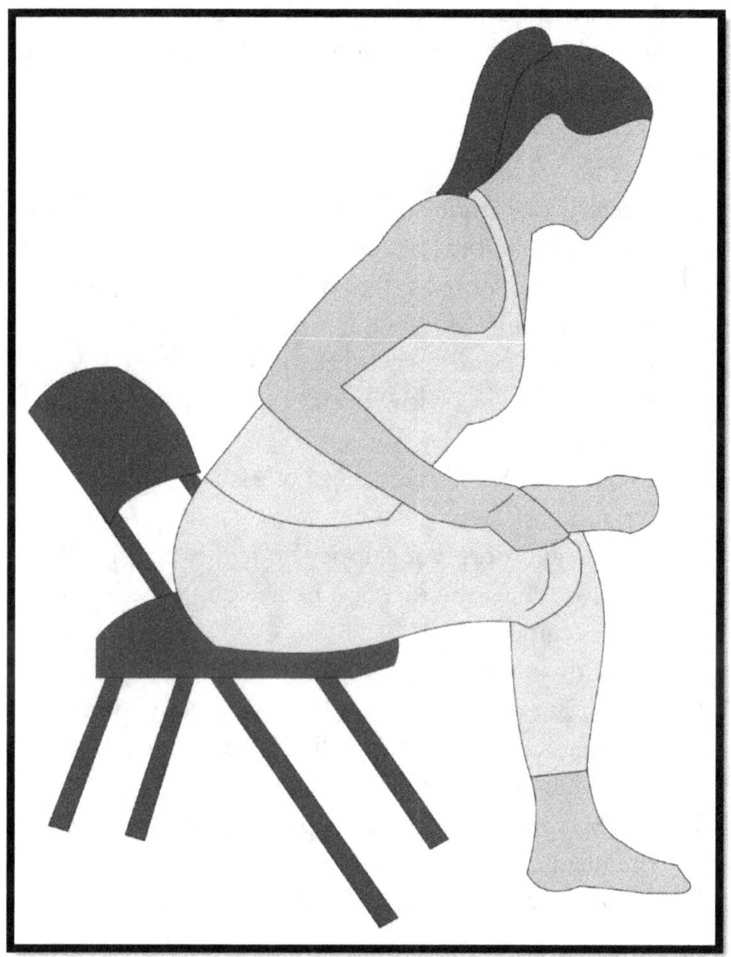

*Effect:*        This exercise helps to stretch the piriformis muscle.

*Start Position:*    Sit tall on the chair, with your thighs supported on the seat, knees hip width distance apart. Place your right ankle over the left knee, making a figure of 4 with the legs.

*Steps:*

1.  Stretch your spine straight in this position trying to free your hip joint as you inhale. Let the right knee go down under the effect of gravity opening the right hip joint.
2.  Exhale and bend forward from this stretched position, leading with your chest while still looking ahead.
3.  Breathe while stretching and release the spine and hip joints slowly.
4.  Exhale and drop your upper body down towards the floor. Feel the increase in stretch in the hip and spine region.
5.  Hold this position for 30 seconds.
6.  Come out of this position by raising your spine up, keeping it straight while still keeping the neck and shoulders relaxed as you inhale.
7.  As the spine comes in the upright position, raise the head and look in front.
8.  Repeat the above sequence on other side.

*Fine Tips:*

1.  Piriformis muscle can be stretched in three different ways. You can choose the technique in which you are most comfortable.

## Lying Down Figure of Four Stretch

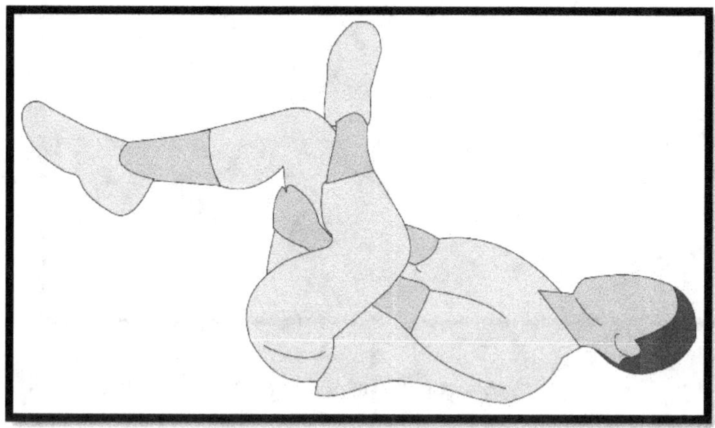

*Effect:*   This exercise helps to stretch the piriformis muscle.

*Start Position:*   Lie on your back, bend your legs and place your feet flat on the ground, hip width distance apart. Place your left ankle over the right knee making a figure of four with your legs.

*Steps:*

1.  Place your right hand behind right knee and gently pull it bringing it towards the chest as you exhale.
2.  Keep pushing the left knee gently away as you pull the right knee, to maintain figure of four.
3.  Hold the stretch where it is comfortable, for 30 seconds. Keep breathing into the stretched muscles, relaxing them.
4.  Gently bring the legs back to start position as you inhale and repeat on the other side.

## Supine Piriformis Stretch

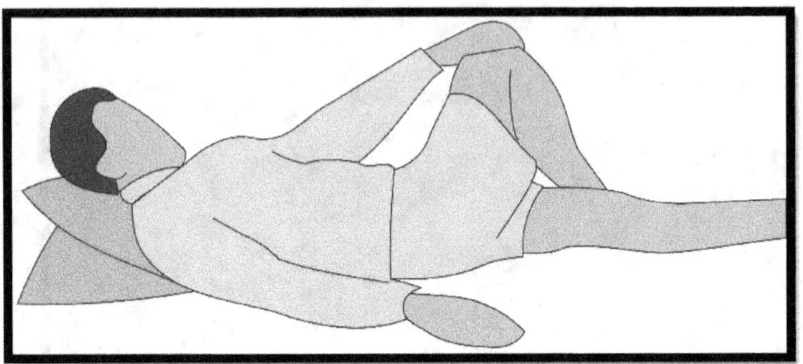

*Effect:*  This exercise helps to stretch the piriformis muscle.

*Start Position:*  Lie down on your back with legs straight.

*Steps:*

1. Bend your right leg and place the right foot flat on the mat by the side of the left knee.
2. Hold the right knee with the left hand and pull it across the midline of the body. Keep the right hip on the floor as you do this.
3. Feel the stretch on the outside of the right leg and hold it for 20-30 seconds.
4. Breathe into the contracted muscles relaxing them.
5. Come back to the start position and repeat with the left leg.

## Buttocks Stretch for Piriformis Muscle

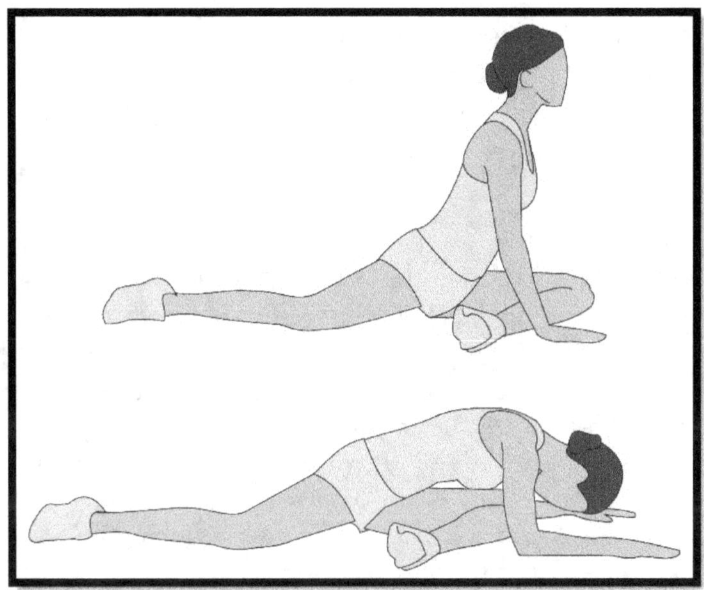

*Effect:* This exercise stretches piriformis muscle.

*Start Position:* Come onto all fours position. Bring the left leg forward, taking the foot across and underneath the body, so that the left knee is outside the body.

*Steps:*

1. Keeping the pelvis squared (in one level) start sliding the back leg behind so that your hips lower down to earth as you exhale.
2. Lean forward on the forearm until deep stretch is felt. Do not forcefully push down the body.
3. Hold the stretch for 20-30 seconds, breathing into the tight muscles relaxing them.

_Fine Tips:_

1. If you feel the stretch too much, you can place a blanket or rolled towel under the hip being stretched and keep your foot flexed to protect the knee.

# QUICK STRETCHING EXERCISES AT WORKPLACE

These stretches have been specially designed to be done in the office. Doing these up to three times a day will help you relax back muscles and decrease the build-up of stress which comes from long hours of sitting. This in turn arrests the onset of back pain and muscle stiffening thus helping you to focus more at your work.

## L Shaped Body Stretch

_Effect:_ Stretches the calves, back, shoulder and arm muscles and relieves tension in the same. Opens up the chest. Frees breathing.

_Start Position:_ Stand straight facing the desk of a height equal to your hip height. The feet should be hip-width distance apart with the outer edges of the feet parallel to each other. The hips & shoulders should be squared (facing forward) and the chin parallel to the floor.

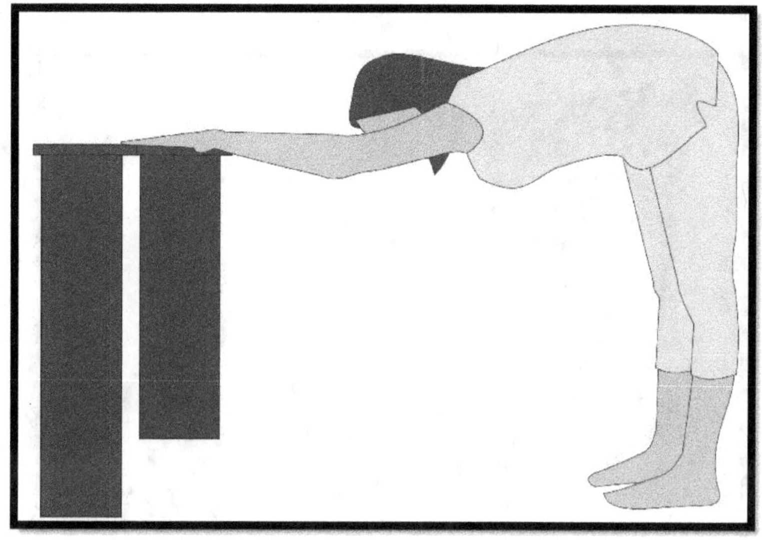

*Steps:*
1.  Bend forward and place your hands on the desk, shoulder-width distance apart, making a 90 degree angle at your hips. Exhale. Keep your neck and head aligned with the spine.
2.  Give a nice stretch to the spine, pulling the tail-bone away from the crown of the head. Hold this position for 30 seconds to 1 minute.
3.  Keep breathing while stretching the calves, hamstrings, back muscles, shoulder muscles & arms and release the stress in them.
4.  Come out of the position by pushing into the hands and then straighten up. Inhale.

*Fine Tips:*
1.  Keep your core involved and use your arms to come out of the stretch position. Using only your back muscles would put undue stress on your spine.

## Forward Bends in Sitting Position

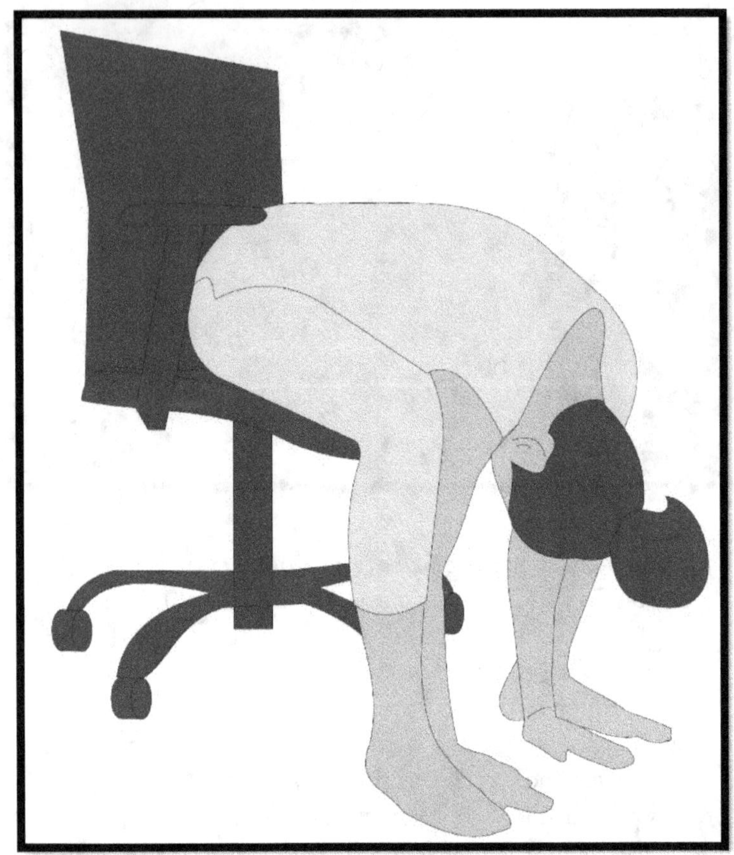

*Effect:*     Stretches the muscles of the back and pelvic region. Relaxes the neck and spine. Reduces tightness of hip muscles thus improving hip joint mobility. Improves posture.

*Start position:*    Sit straight with feet grounded and placed at a distance little wider than the hip width distance. Knees should be directly over the ankles and toes rotated slightly outwards.

*Steps:*
1. Place your hands on mid-thigh & stretch your spine. Inhale.
2. Keeping your feet firm, push into the feet; bend your body, vertebrae by vertebrae from the hip region to chest till your hands reach the floor. Exhale.
3. Release your shoulder, neck and head towards the floor. Keep breathing into the hip sockets, spine, shoulders & neck as you relax them. Hold for 30 seconds to 1 minute.
4. Come out of this position by uncurling your lower back first, followed by upper back, then neck & finally straighten your head as you push through the feet into the floor.
5. This exercise can be repeated often throughout the day.

*Fine Tips:*
1. Sit on a rolled up towel placed on a chair, in case of hip tightness.
2. Always keep the feet firmly on the ground for good balance as you relax your joints and muscles.
3. If your hands don't reach the floor as you bend down, place them over some piled up books or files and relax.

Seated Spine Twists

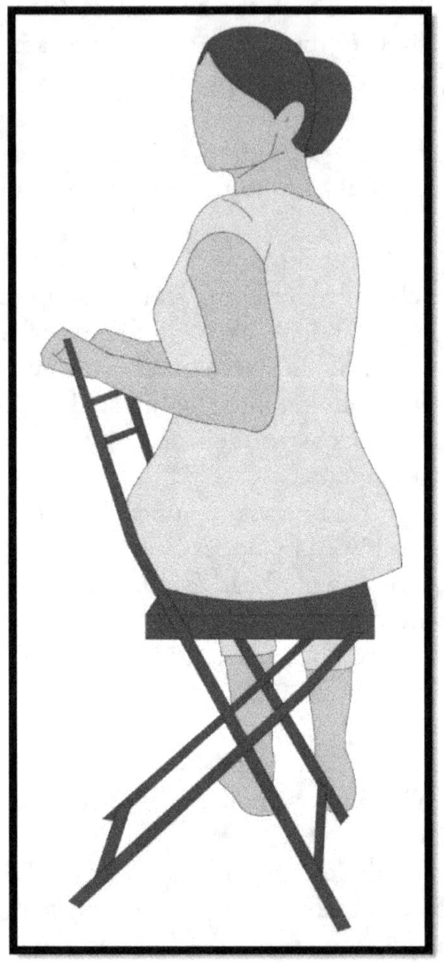

*Effect:*     Stretches the lower back, upper back, shoulder and neck muscles, releasing tension from the same. Stretches the front and sides of the body. Improves breathing & posture.

*Start Position:*    Sit sideways on the chair with thigh parallel to the back of the chair. Sit straight with chin parallel to the floor, shoulders relaxed and spine tall. The legs should make an angle of 90 degrees at the hips, knees and ankles. The feet should be hip-width distance apart. Distribute weight equally between both buttocks.

*Steps:*
1. From the side sitting position (left thigh next to the chair back), start turning towards the back of the chair.
2. Inhale as you stretch your spine straight from the tail-bone to the crown of the head and exhale as you turn. Keep stretching and turning till you hold the back of the chair.
3. Look behind over your left shoulder in the final position. Keep breathing into the stretch. Hold this position for 30 seconds to 1 minute.
4. Turn your torso back to the start position as you exhale.
5. Repeat the whole sequence on the Opposite side, sitting with right thigh next to the back of the chair.
6. This stretch can be repeated often throughout the day.

*Fine Tips:*
1. Stretch your spine straight while inhaling and turn while exhaling, giving a nice squeezing action to your torso.

## Standing Side Bends

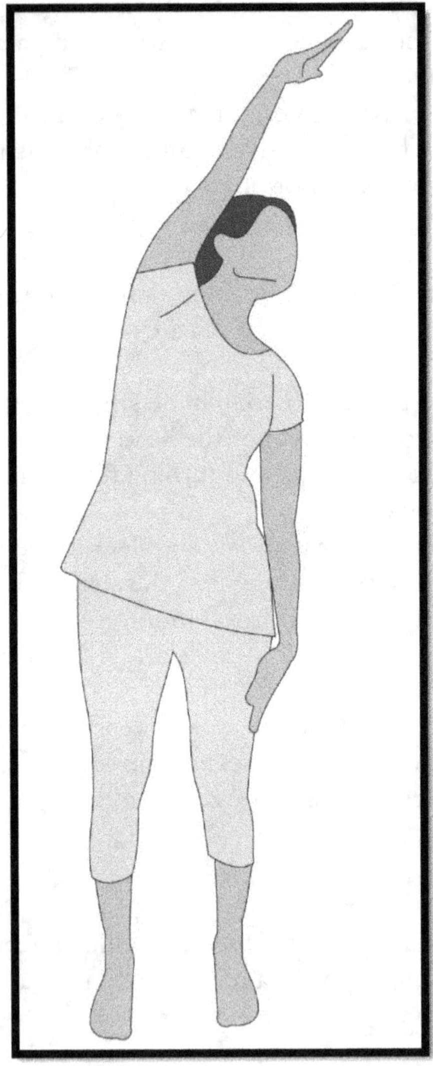

*Effect:*        Stretches the arms and sides of the body. Releases stress in the stretching body parts. Improves posture.

*Start Position:*   Stand tall with feet hip-width distance apart and outer edges of the feet parallel to each other. Tuck in your naval and contract your thighs and gluteal muscles. Keep the shoulders relaxed, chest broad and chin parallel to the floor.

*Steps:*
1.  Raise your right arm up with the palm facing the left side.
2.  Stretch the right arm up, giving a nice stretch to the right side of the trunk. Keep the weight equally distributed between both feet as you stretch. Inhale.
3.  Bend towards the left side with your right fingertips trying to reach towards the ceiling diagonally. Exhale. Feel the increase in stretch on the right side of the trunk.
4.  Breathe into the stretch. Hold for 5 counts and relax.
5.  Come back to the start position.
6.  Repeat for the left side.
7.  Repeat 2 times for each side.

*Fine Tips:*
1.  Keep your weight equally distributed between both feet, pushing into the foot of the stretching side as you bend towards the other side.

## Standing Backwards Bend

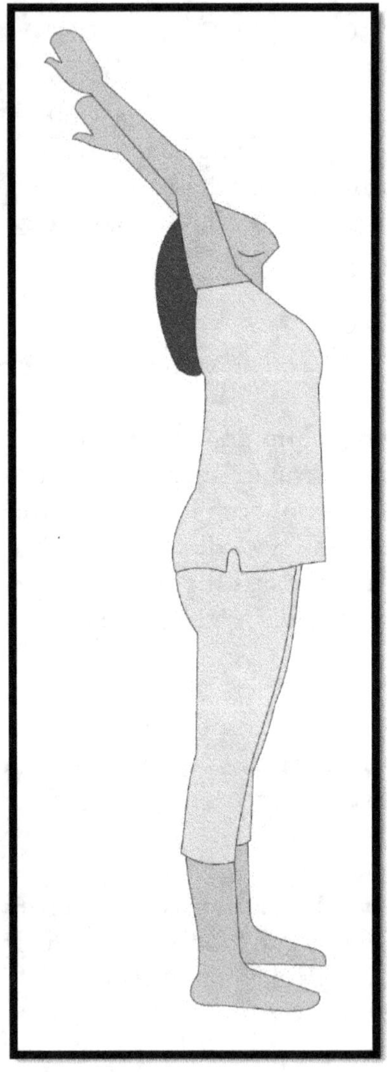

_Effect:_  Stretches the front side of your body. Improves posture. Extends the spine, thus preventing a hunched back. Frees up breathing.

_Start Position:_  Stand tall with feet hip-Width distance apart and outer edges of the feet parallel to each other. The thighs should be contracted, gluteal muscles tight and navel tucked in. The shoulders should be relaxed, chest broad and chin parallel to the floor.

_Steps:_
1.  Raise your arms up, with shoulders pulled down maintaining distance between arms & ears. Inhale.
2.  Bend at your upper back, with the finger tips reaching towards the ceiling. Exhale.
3.  Feel the stretch on the front side of your body, shoulders and upper back. Keep breathing into the stretches as you pull yourself up and back.
4.  Hold here for 5 counts and relax. Keep deep breathing.
5.  Come back to start position as you exhale.
6.  Repeat twice.

_Fine Tips:_
1.  Keep weight distribution between both feet equal for the entire duration of stretching.

# CHAPTER 8

# Management of Acute / Chronic Back Pain in case of Exaggerated Lumbar Curve

Exaggerated lumbar curve is associated with Anterior Pelvic Tilt wherein the pelvic bone tilts forward and the butt juts out at the back. While this may be considered enhancing the sex appeal (especially for females) in certain cultures, the unnatural tilt puts extra pressure on the lower back and may lead to severe back pain for the individuals.

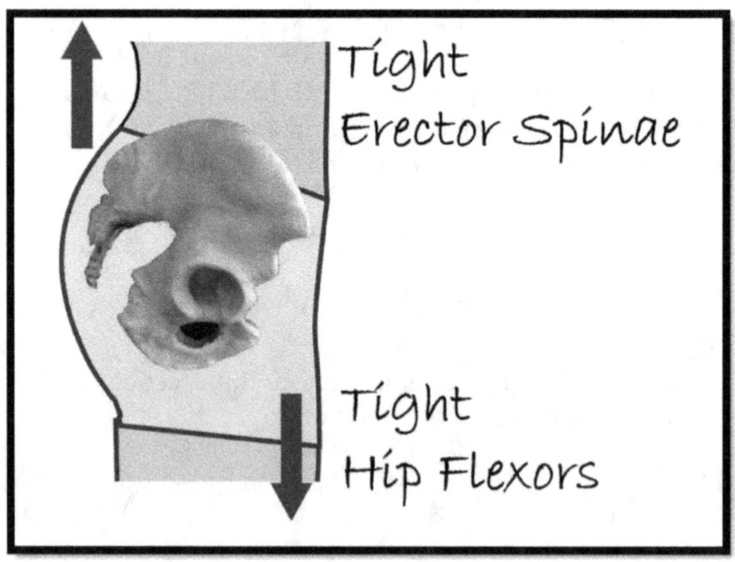


The most common cause of anterior pelvic tilt is incorrect sitting for long hours. A sedentary lifestyle, especially among people who spend long hours sitting in a desk job, prolonged sitting posture puts unnatural pressure on the back and thigh muscles. The hip flexors and low back extensors become tight while abdominals & gluteal muscles get weak. This muscle imbalance leads to adaptation of pelvic bones to maintain bodily balance leading to chronic anterior pelvic tilt, which leads to an exaggerated lumbar curve.

To manage the lower back pain caused by this situation, we need to strengthen the core, mobilize and stretch the tight muscles (hip flexors and low back extensors) and strengthen the weak muscles (abdominals and gluteals).

You should do the following exercises thrice a week.

| | Exercise | Page |
|---|---|---|
| 1 | Pelvic Tilt (Back Imprinting) | 41 |
| 2 | Back Imprinting with One Leg Raise | 42 |
| 3 | Back Imprinting with One Leg Raise 2" | 44 |
| 4 | Back Imprinting with One Knee to Chest | 45 |
| 5 | Back Imprinting with Knees Pressing on the Ball | 47 |
| 6 | Back Imprinting with Heel Slide | 48 |
| 7 | Bridging with Arms by Side of Body | 49 |
| 8 | Single Leg Raise in Prone | 58 |
| 9 | Back Imprinting with Arms and Legs raise and Partial Sit-up | 68 |
| 10 | Abdominal Crunch on Physio Ball | 76 |
| 11 | Side Abdominal Crunches | 77 |

# CHAPTER 9

# Management of Acute / Chronic Back Pain in case of Flattened Lumbar Curve

Flattened lumbar curve is associated with Posterior Pelvic Tilt wherein the pelvic bone tilts backward. This tilt occurs due to contraction of the hip extensors and the straight abdominal muscles.

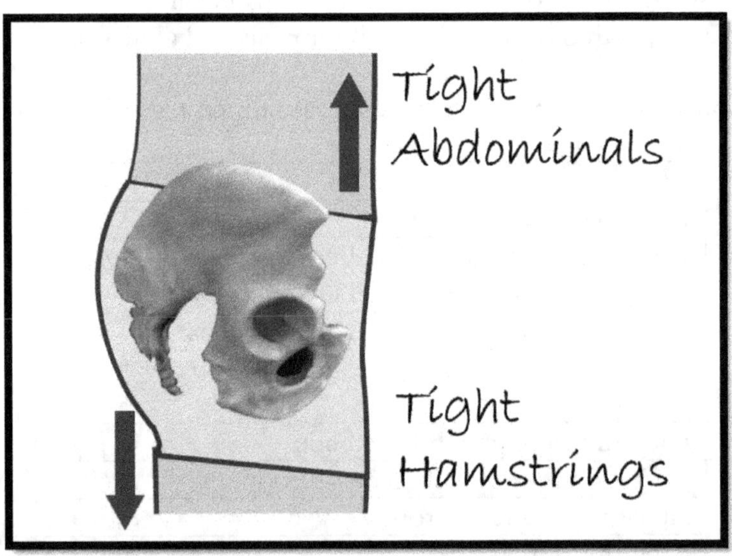


The most common cause of Posterior pelvic tilt are poor sitting/standing postures (having a slouched back), lifting/carrying weight or poor sleeping posture. An incorrect exercise regime can also lead to posterior pelvic tilt. An exercise routine focusing on strengthening of gluteals, abdominals and hamstrings predominantly may lead to posterior pelvic tilt if the back muscles are not strong enough to counterbalance the targeted muscles.

## Lying Face Down on Abdomen

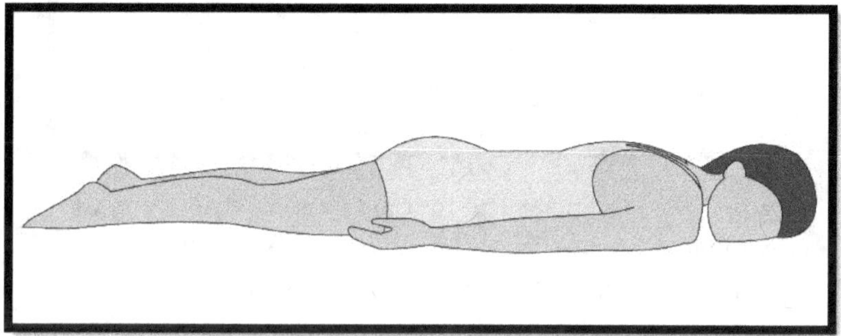

*Effect:*        This is the first aid exercise for acute and chronic back pain.

*Start Position:*    Lie face down straight with your arms by the side of your body and head turned to one side.

*Steps:*

1.  Take deep breaths and relax in this position for 2-3 minutes trying to remove all the tension from muscles in your back.

*Fine Tips:*

1.  This exercise should be done once at the beginning of each exercise session with sessions spread evenly six to eight times a day.

## Extension on Forearm from Face Down Lying on Abdomen

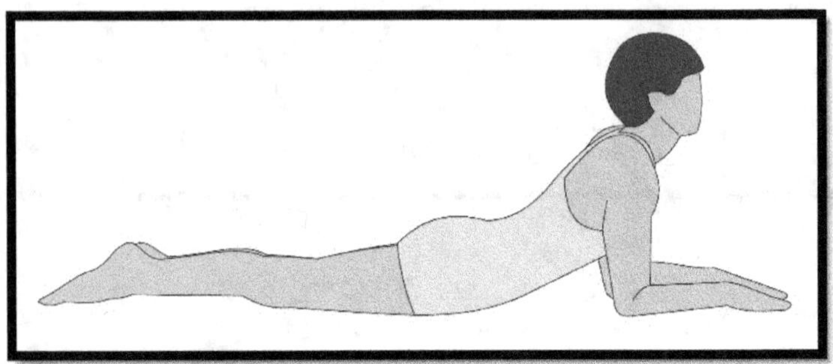

*Effect:* This is the first aid exercise for acute and chronic low back pain & should be done after the exercise mentioned above (i.e. Lying Face Down on Abdomen).

*Start Position:* Lie face down straight on your abdomen, place your elbows under your shoulders and prop yourself up on forearms.

*Steps:*

1. Take deep breaths in this position, trying to relax the tense back muscles.
2. Hold this position for 2 to 3 minutes.
3. Slowly return to the starting position.
4. Should be repeated six to eight times a day, spread evenly throughout the day

*Fine Tips:*

1. In case the pain increases while attempting this exercise, modified extension exercise should be done.

Extension on Hands from Face Down Lying On Abdomen

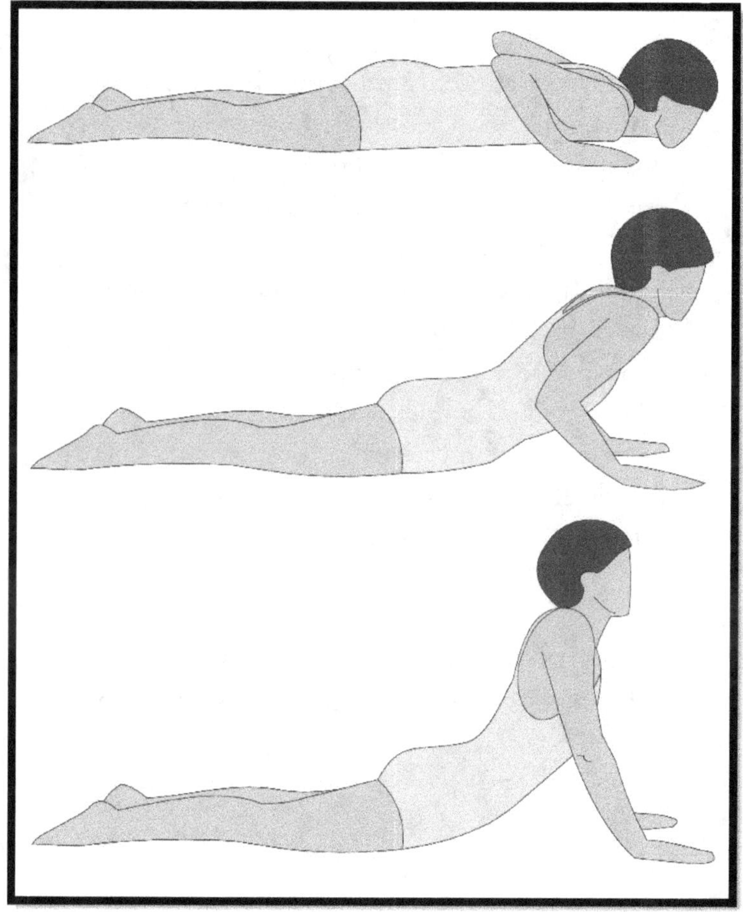

*Effect:*          This is the most affective first aid procedure in treatment of acute low back pain and stiffness.

*Start Position:*   Remain face down and place your hands under your shoulders.

*Steps:*

1. Push yourself up from this position as much as the pain permits.
2. Relax your pelvis, hips and legs as you do this movement, keeping them hanging limp and allowing the back to sag.
3. Hold this position for 1-2 seconds and slowly lower yourself down to the starting position.
4. Slowly return to the starting position.
5. The above mentioned movement should be performed 10 times each session trying to increase the extension range as the pain permits.
6. Do 6-8 sessions per day spread evenly.

*Fine Tips:*

1. In case of no response or increasing pain on attempting this exercise, modified extension should be done.

## Extension in Standing

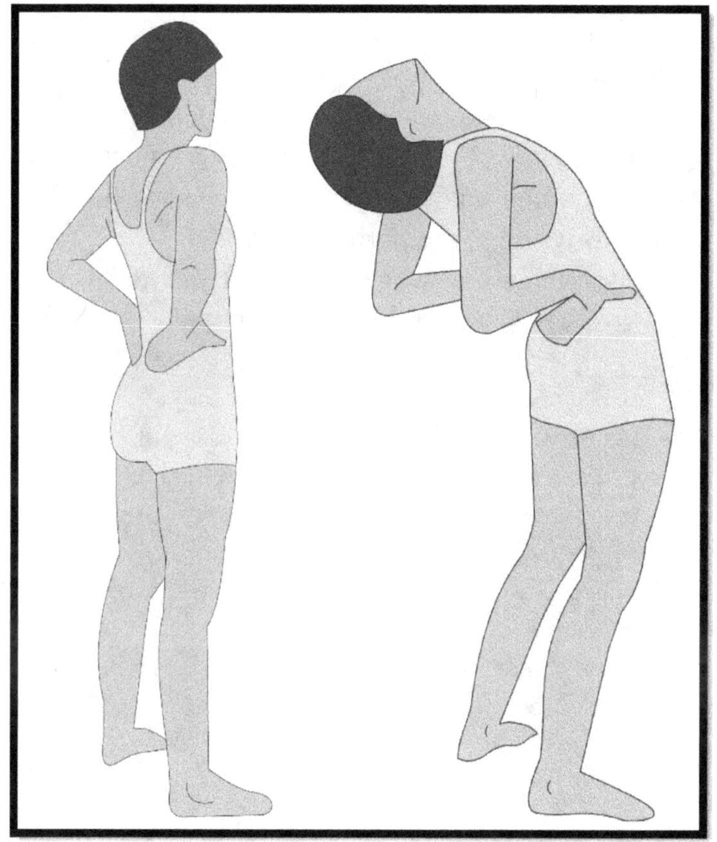

*Effect:* Stretches the abdominals, hence helps in correcting the Posterior Pelvic Tilt.

*Start Position:* Stand tall with your feet hip width distance apart. Place your hands on your waist with your fingers pointing backwards.

*Steps:*

1. Using hands as a fulcrum, bend your trunk backwards at the waist as far as you can within pain limits.
2. Keep your knees straight as you do this movement.
3. Maintain the bent position for 1-2 secs and then slowly return to the starting position.
4. Repeat this movement 8-10 times, trying to increase the backward bend each time.

*Fine Tips:*

1. This exercise can be performed in place of earlier exercise (Extension on Hands from Face Down Lying on Abdomen), if extension from lying position is not possible.
2. This can be used as a preventive measure towards recurrence of low back pain.
3. Repeat the exercise as and when possible when you want a break from working in forward bend position.

## Leg Flexion from Lying Down on Back

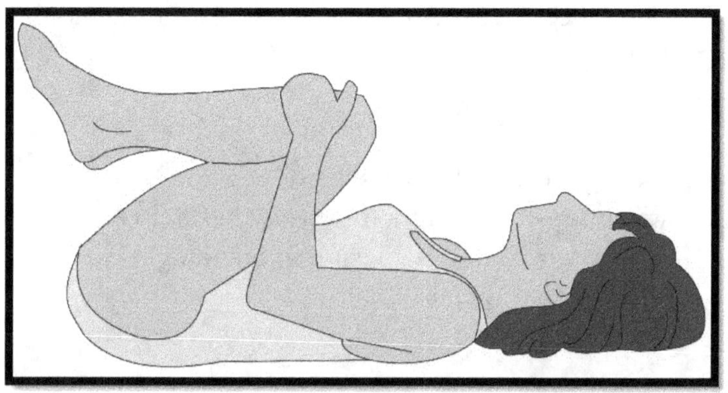

*Effect:* This exercise helps to stretch the damaged tissues which might have shortened or become less flexible during healing.

*Start Position:* Lie down straight on your back with knees bent and feet flat on the floor or bed.

*Steps:*

1. Bring both knees up towards the chest.
2. Pull the knees as close to the chest as pain permits with hands placed behind the knees.
3. Maintain this position for a second or two and then slowly lower down your legs returning to the start position.
4. Keep your head on the floor / bed and legs bent at knees throughout the exercise.
5. Try to pull your knees little closer to the chest with every repetition trying to reach the maximum possible degree of flexion.

6. Repeat this exercise 5-6 times per session.
7. Do 2-4 sessions per day equally spread throughout the day.

*Fine Tips:*

1. Once you are able to easily pull the knees to chest without pain, progress to next two exercises (Flexion in Sitting & Flexion in Standing).

## Flexion in Sitting

*Effect:* Stretches the muscles of lower back and pelvic region. Reduces tightness of hip muscles thus improving hip joint mobility.

*Start Position:* Sit at the edge of a steady chair with your knees and feet slightly more than hip width apart and your hands resting between your legs.

*Steps:*

1. Bend your trunk forward, leading with your heart and try to touch the floor with your hands in this position. Do not curve your upper back.
2. Return immediately to the start position.
3. Do 5-6 repetitions per session trying to increase the bend at each cycle reaching the maximum possible degree of flexion during the session.

4. Do 2-4 sessions per day equally spread throughout the day.

*Fine Tips:*

1. You can make room for the bend by successively bending your elbows and then reaching out to the base of the chair as your range of motion improves.

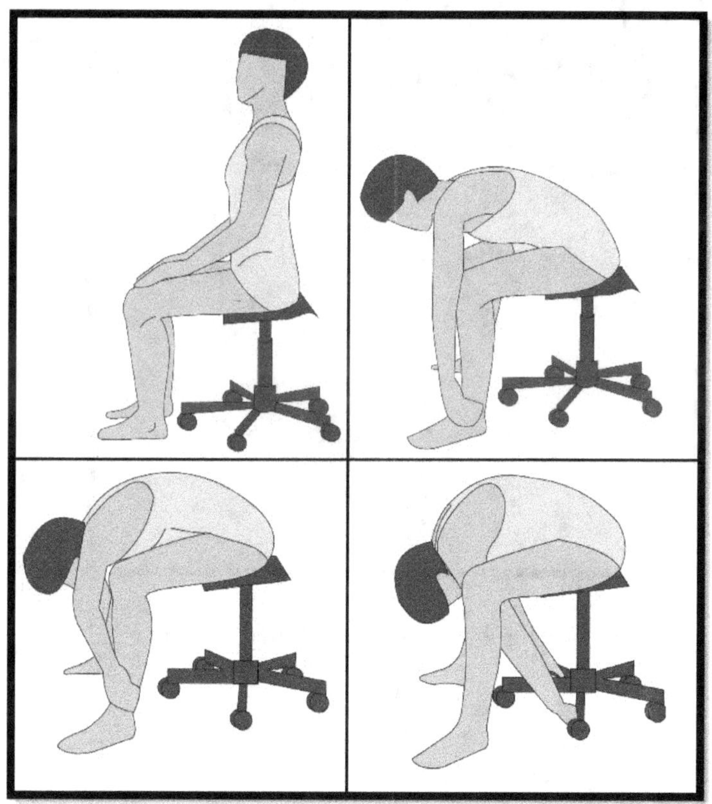

## Flexion in Standing

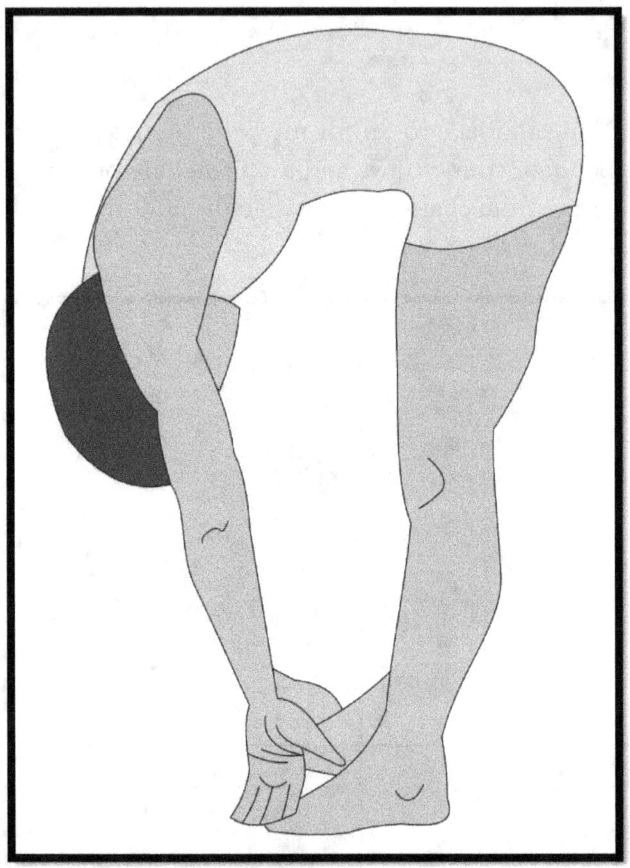

*Effect:*   Stretches the back, gluteals, hamstrings and calf muscles.

*Start Position:*   Stand tall with feet hip width apart and your hands by the side of body.

*Steps:*

1. Bend forward, running your fingers down your legs as far as you can comfortable reach.
2. Return to the start position.
3. Do 5-6 repetitions per session trying to increase the bend at each cycle reaching the maximum possible degree of flexion during the session.
4. Do 2-4 sessions per day equally spread throughout the day.

The exercises 1 to 3 are first aids and can be performed at the first sign of back pain. Nevertheless if the person is not able to move at all, then 2 days' bed rest along with self-care techniques for back ache should be taken before starting the exercises. Exercises 1-3 should be repeated for at least 1 week during which centralization of the pain (i.e. the pain should become more localized in the centre of back) should occur. Attention about the posture and movement should be taken all the times avoiding slouch sitting or standing positions.

The flexion exercise should be started 2 weeks after pain free completion of extension exercises.

In case the pain does not reduce or increases with these exercises then modified extension exercises should be performed.

*Modified Extension Exercises in No Relief of Pain*

## Lying Face Down on Abdomen with Hip Shifted Away from Pain Site

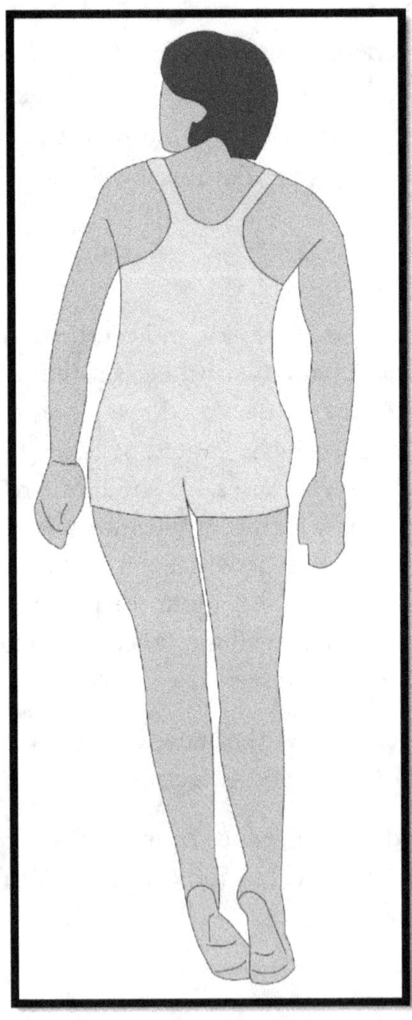



Lying Face Down on Abdomen with Hip Shifted
Away from Pain Site

_Effect:_     This is the first aid exercise for acute and chronic back pain which does not go with straight extension.

_Start Position:_   Lie face down straight with your arms by the side of your body and head turned to one side.

_Steps:_

1.  Shift your hip away from the pain site.
2.  Take deep breaths and relax in this position for 2-3 minutes trying to remove all the tension from muscles in your back.

_Fine Tips:_

1.  This exercise should be done once at the beginning of each exercise session with sessions spread evenly six to eight times a day.

## Extension on Forearm from Face Down on Abdomen with Hip Shifted Away from Pain Site

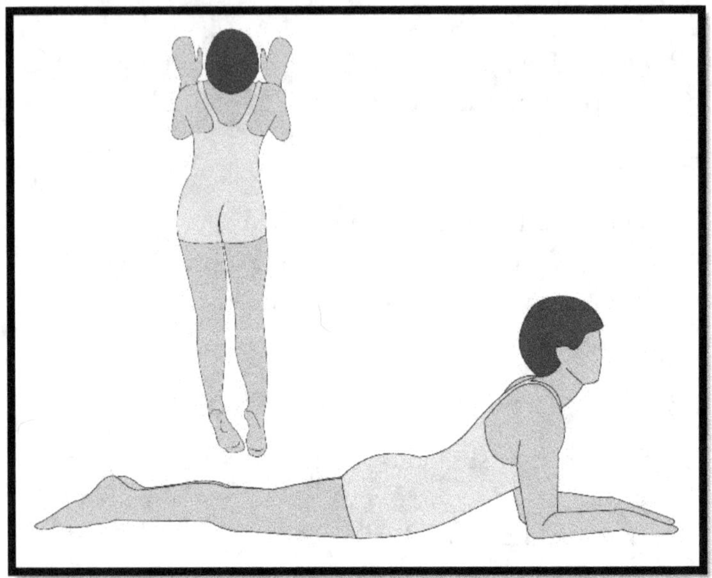

*Effect:*   This is the first aid exercise for acute and chronic low back pain which should be done after the ex no 1 mentioned above.

*Start Position:*   Lie face down on your abdomen with the hips shifted away from the pain site.

*Steps:*

1.  Place your elbows under your shoulders and prop yourself up on forearms.
2.  Take deep breaths in this position, letting the back sag and hips, pelvis and legs relax in this position.
3.  Hold this position for 2 to 3 minutes.

4.  Slowly return to the starting position.

5.  Should be repeated six to eight times a day, spread evenly throughout the day.

# Extension on Arm from Face Down on Abdomen with Hip Shifted Away from Pain Site

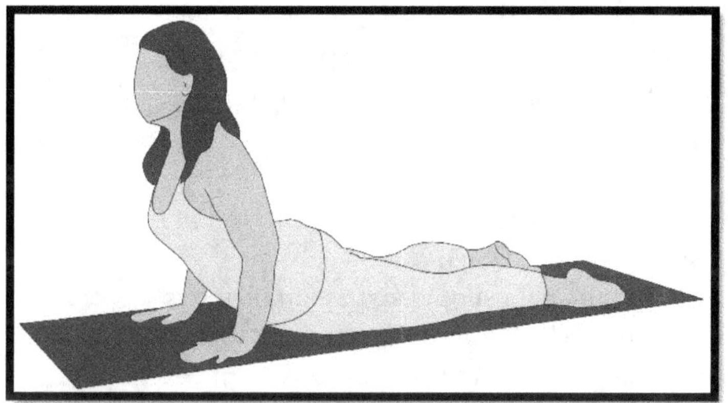

*Effect:*　　　　This is the most affective first aid procedure in treatment of acute low back pain and stiffness.

*Start Position:*　Lie down in face down position with your hips shifted away from pain site and hands placed under your shoulders.

*Steps:*

1.  Push yourself up from this position as much as the pain permits.

2.  Relax your pelvis, hips and legs as you do this movement, keeping them hanging limp and allowing the back to sag.
3.  Hold this position for 1-2 seconds and slowly lower yourself down to the starting position.
4.  Slowly return to the starting position.
5.  The above mentioned movement should be performed 10 times each session trying to increase the extension range as the pain permits.
6.  Do 6-8 sessions per day spread evenly.

A slight increase in pain is expected with the start of extension exercises, which should subside after 5-6 sessions and the pain should start centralizing to a specific spot on your back. In case of increase or spreading of pain to a wider area after couple of sessions of the exercises, you should stop performing these exercises and consult your doctor or physical therapist.

You can start with the both legs flexion from the lying on back position, as mentioned above, 2 weeks after the pain free completion of extension from modified position, to decrease stiffness in the back. A slight increase in pain in low back is expected on start of this exercise due to stretching of shortened structures in the back. But this pain should subside with repetition of the exercise.

In case increase or peripheralization of pain after couple of sessions of the exercises you should stop doing flexion exercises and continue with extensions

*Pain Reduction or Centralisation of Back Pain- Indicating Improvements of the Factors Causing Back Pain*

Once you have designed your back-pain exercise regime (as described in upcoming chapter), you need to be sure that the chosen exercises are helping you to improve your back condition and not worsening it. You need to look for one of the following effects to be sure that exercises, movements and postures chosen are correcting the distortion or bulging that may have developed in the joints of the lower back.

a. There is reduction in intensity and eventually termination of pain, after doing the exercises.

b. There is increase or decrease of intensity of pain or change of location of pain following the initiation of exercises but eventually reduction of pain and finally cessation of pain completely after few sessions.

c. There is centralisation of pain, immediately or after couple of exercise sessions. Centralisation of pain means, the pain moves from peripheral parts of body like legs, buttocks or thighs to the midline (spine) or low back and localises there. Eventually the pain ceases to exist after a few sessions.

The pain may initially increase as you start with any exercise, but eventually as you continue with the exercises it should come down at least to the former level after 1-2 sessions and then finally reduce and centralise in 3-4 days and disappear after 1-3 weeks. If the symptoms were present for weeks or months, the response to the exercise might take 10-14 days.

*When Should You Stop Continuing the Exercises and Consult a Doctor or Physical Therapist?*

The pain may increase or change its location after starting with certain sets of exercise. If the increased intensity of pain does not reduce after 2-3 sessions, (i.e. by the next day), or you feel the pain moving to the buttocks, thighs or limbs, that is further away from back, immediately stop the exercises.

# CHAPTER 10

## Design your Treatment Plan

In the previous chapters, we have seen the structure of back, the kind of problems that can happen with the lower back, possible causes for these issues and the most effective exercises that you can do to bring relief to a sore back. All the exercises have specific effects (as mentioned along each one) and may not be required in your particular situation. Now we look at how to decide on your individual exercise regime

First and foremost, notice if the pain is persistent during rest as well as while moving (i.e. nerve and tissues are involved) or does it increase with the movement and relieves on rest (i.e. pain is mechanical). If it is the former, then meet your doctor at the first instance. Involvement of nerves strongly indicates issues with the vertebra.

If the pain is mechanical, calibrate the intensity of pain on the scale of 0-10 where grade 10 is intense pain restricting movement of body and 0 is no pain with normal movement of the body.

Check yourself in the mirror for your lumbar curve. Is it exaggerated?

## 8-10 Grade Pain (Very Intense Pain Preventing Movements or Normal Routine)

Take 2 days' bedrest and start with first aid self-management techniques to relieve back pain (see Chapter 4). Our first target is to bring the pain within bearable limits so that you can do the recommended exercises.

## 3-8 Grade Pain (Moderate to Intense Pain While Moving or Doing Daily Activities)

Take heat therapy to mobilize the muscles and provide pain relief to the affected area. Start with Myofascial Release (see Chapter 5). In case of Normal or Exaggerated lumbar curve, do the imprinting exercises in Chapter 6. However in case of a flattened lumbar curve, do the extension exercises followed by flexion exercises as outlined in Chapter 9.

## 1-3 Grade Pain (Very Minimal Pain at Rest, or While Moving or While Doing Routine Activities)

Start with Myofascial Release Exercises (see Chapter 5). Do easy exercises (see Chapter 6) to strengthen the back. Finish with stretching exercises (see Chapter 7).

Once your back feels strong enough after doing 1 month of easy exercises to strengthen the back you can proceed to medium strengthening exercise. 2 months after successful completion of medium strengthening back exercises, you can proceed to advanced strengthening exercise regimes.

The exercise routine should always start with MFR followed by strengthening exercises and end with the stretching exercises.

CHAPTER 11

# Deep Relaxation with Sectional Breathing – An Effective Way to Release Chronic Stress and thus Manage Chronic Back Pain

Deep relaxation works wonders to decrease chronic stress and its effects. When your body is relaxed, it exerts a calming and stabilizing influence on you mind. When your mind is relaxed, it exerts a powerful, tranquilizing and relaxing effect on your body. When both mind and body are relaxed, stress is released and healing occurs.

One of the best ways to counter everyday stresses is to practice sectional breathing. To practice that, follow the following sequence of breathing.

1. <u>Abdominal (Diaphragmatic) breathing</u> –

   a. Place your hands on your abdominal region.
   b. Inhale deeply & slowly. Your abdomen bulges out with inhalation. Hold your breath for few seconds.
   c. Exhale slowly and completely. Your abdomen is drawn inwards continuously and slowly with exhalation.
   d. Before inhaling again, hold your breath.
   e. Repeat this breath cycle 9 times.

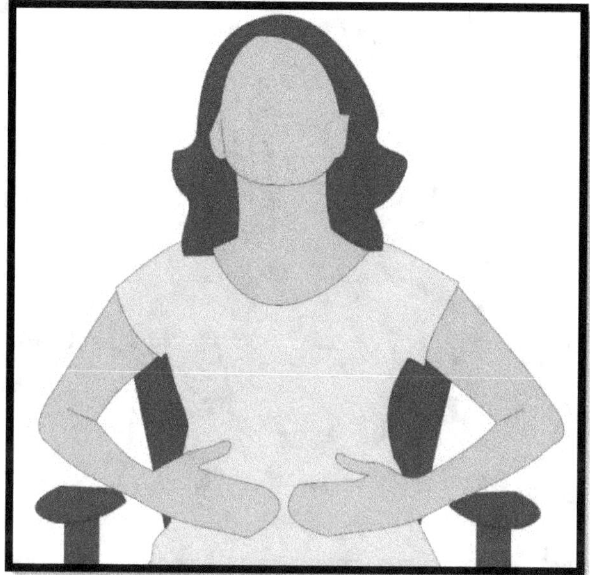

There should be no jerks in the whole process. The breathing should be slow, continuous and relaxed.

2. <u>Thoracic (Intercostal) breathing –</u>
   a. Place your hands on the ribs with the tips of the middle finger touching each other.
   b. Inhale deeply and slowly. While inhaling you should feel the chest cage expanding outwards and upwards. The middle finger tips should move apart a little with inhalation.
   c. Exhale slowly and completely. While exhaling relax the chest wall and return to the starting position, with the chest cage moving backwards, inwards & downwards.

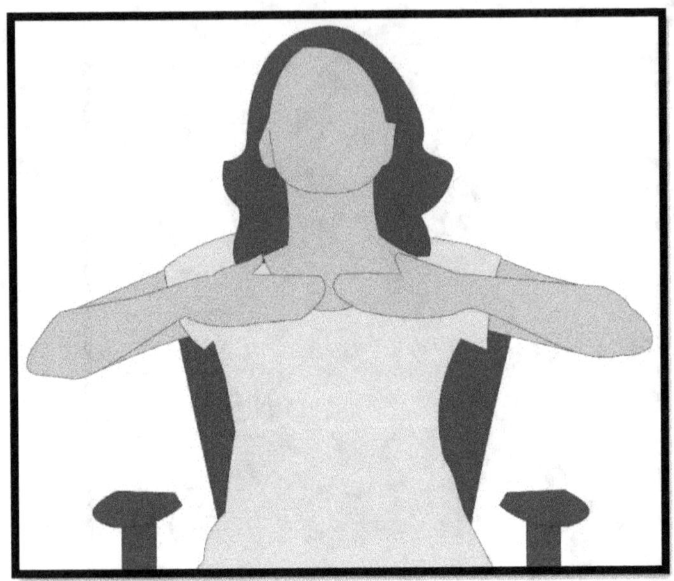

    d.   Repeat this breathing cycle 9 times. There should be no jerks in the whole process. The breathing should be slow, continuous and relaxed.

3.   <u>Clavicular breathing</u> –
    a.   Place your hands on the clavicular region (collar bone).
    b.   Inhale deeply and slowly. While inhaling you should feel your collar bones rising upwards and ahead.
    c.   Exhale slowly and completely. While exhaling you should feel your collar bones and shoulders dropping down to the start position.

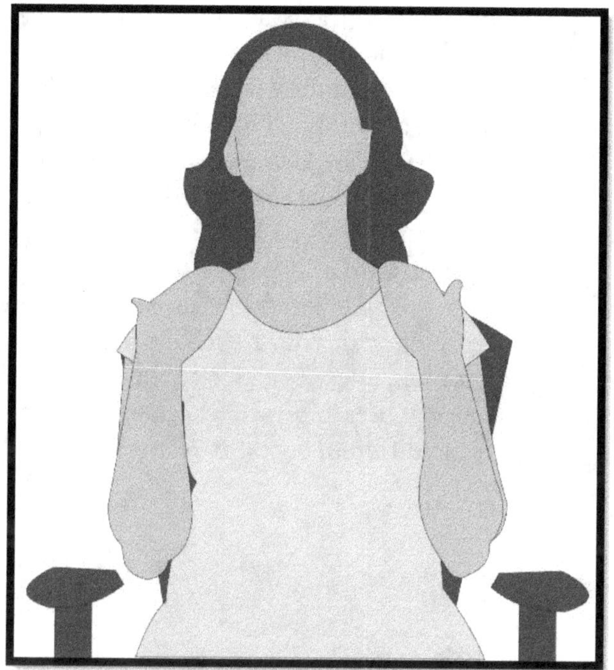

d.   Repeat this breathing cycle 9 times. There should be no jerks in the whole process. The breathing should be slow, continuous and relaxed.

4.   <u>Complete / Full breathing –</u>

This is the combination of abdomen, thoracic & clavicular breathing.

a.   Sit in a comfortable position; Start inhaling in the sequence of abdomen, chest & clavicle. Your abdomen should bulge, chest cage should expand forward, outward &

upwards and the collarbone should get raised ahead & upwards.

b.  Now exhale in the sequence of clavicle, chest & abdomen. The collarbone should move backward & downwards, the chest cage should move backwards, inwards & downwards and the abdomen should get drawn inwards.

c.  Once you have practiced enough of guided breathing with your hands on the abdomen, chest & clavicle, you can practice sectional breathing anywhere by focusing on the different sections respectively.

# CHAPTER 12

## Alternative Back Ache Treatments

Alternative back pain treatments are unlike traditional western medical standard treatments, but may be as effective as the later. Following are some of the most prominent ones.

### Manual Manipulations

This includes physical adjustment done to the spine by a chiro practitioner or other healthcare provider. Hand thrust of varying speed and force are applied to the spinal structure to improve mobility, decrease stiffness and reduce pain or discomfort.

### Acupuncture

Acupuncture is a form of Chinese medicine. Acupuncture is based on the theory that body contains pattern of energy flow which is referred to as *qi* (pronounced as *chi*) and proper flow of *qi* is considered to decrease pain and discomfort in the body. In acupuncture, hair thin needles are inserted at acupuncture points in specific combinations in the skin, correcting the flow of *qi*. These needles stay in the body for about an hour. Acupuncture has shown to provide pain relief in many people.

*Massage Therapy*

Massage therapy can be used as an effective adjunct to low back pain treatments.

Massage improves the blood circulation in the affected area, thus increasing the oxygen and nutrient supply in the area. Lack of oxygen in the affected area is the main cause of increased lactic acid production and thus soreness after physical activity. With massage the lactic acid is drained out thus decreasing soreness.

Massage relaxes muscles for improved range of motion. Muscle relaxation also helps to treat insomnia. Massage increases the endorphin levels in the body. Endorphins are the chemicals that make you feel good, which is effective in managing lower back pain.

*Mindful Yoga & Meditation*

Yoga is a group of physical, mental and spiritual practices that originated in ancient India. It is a mind-body workout that combines strengthening and stretching poses with deep breathing and meditation or relaxation. Yoga can help by healing injured muscles, speeding time to recover from injury, prevent re-injury and helping to maintain a regular level of daily activities and avoid disability.

In general most yoga postures are safe in low back pain. However, in case of severe or chronic lower back pain, a detailed evaluation and accurate diagnosis should be done by a health care professional before starting yoga.

*Benefits of Yoga for Back*

1. Muscle Strengthening:  Holding some positions and doing movements in those positions in yoga help to strengthen muscles of back and abdominal muscles. Back and abdominal muscles are the main muscles supporting spine, thus helping body to maintain a proper upright posture and movement. When these muscles are well conditioned it helps to prevent lower back pain.

2. Stretching & Relaxation: Yoga incorporates stretching and relaxation, which helps to reduce the tension in stress carrying muscles. You need to hold yoga posture for 10-60 seconds. During holding the posture still, some muscles are stretching and others flexing. Thus these postures help to relax as well as improve the flexibility of the body, reducing low back pain. With yoga stretches, the blood flow in the area increases, increasing the supply of oxygen and nutrients in the area and also increasing the flow out of toxins. This improves the overall nourishment of the muscle, soft tissue and the joints in the low back. Deep, slow, controlled, rhythmic breathing through nose is very important while stretching in the yoga postures. Deep inhalation and exhalation

helps to relax the stretched muscles better, thus relieving low back pain.

3.  <u>Posture, Balance & Body Alignment</u>: In yoga postures, your body has to be in the perfect alignment to sustain a stance or add movements to the posture. This brings good balance in your body as you are stretching and strengthening through the posture. Your spine, head, shoulders and hips are properly aligned. Proper alignment and good posture with spine in natural, neutral curve is the key requirement to prevent and rectify low back pain.

4.  <u>Body Awareness</u>: Getting into various postures and maintaining them gives you as insight into which positions are feasible for you to do and what are your limitations. With this increased awareness you can take preventive measures as to what type of motions you should and should not do.

5.  <u>Psychological & Emotional Well Being</u>: Meditation and sustaining yoga postures bring a calmness and stability in your mind and body. This helps to dissipate anxiety and stress. The increased oxygen supply which occurs after breathing exercises (*Pranayama*) helps to maintain a rhythm in your mind and body.

# Bonus

I hope you liked the book and have already started doing these exercises. To make it easier for you to follow these exercises, here is some bonus material.

You can download an easy to use chart of these exercises, which can be used for quick reference. Placed at a prominent place in your home, this would also serve as a handy reminder to do your exercises at regular interval.

**https://www.fitness-sutra.com/go?id=141150**

SCAN ME! 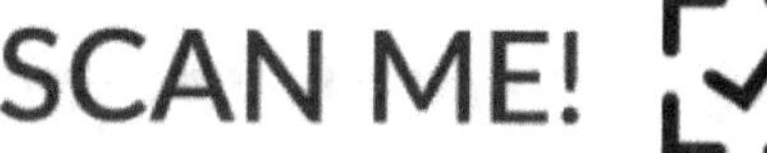 

You can also subscribe to my mailing list to get more tips & motivation to do these exercises.

Your feedback would help me improve this book. Please give me a review on

**https://www.fitness-sutra.com/go?id=141207**

 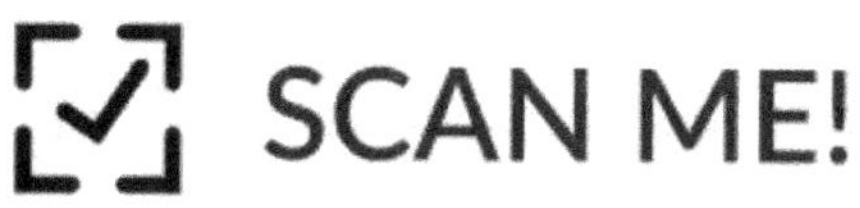 SCAN ME!

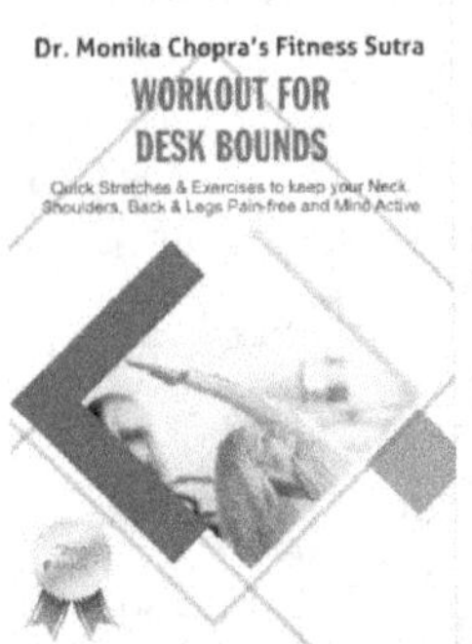


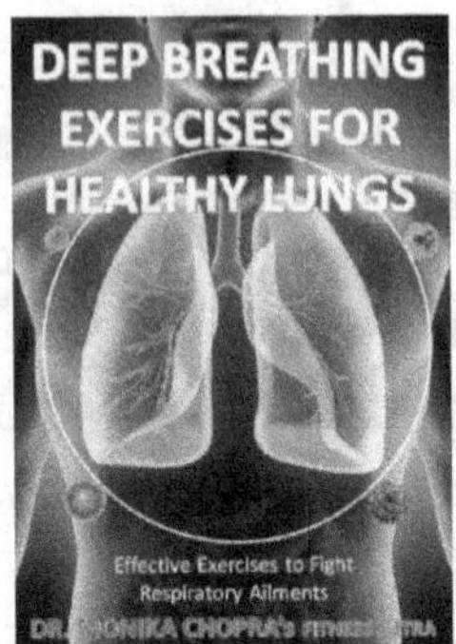


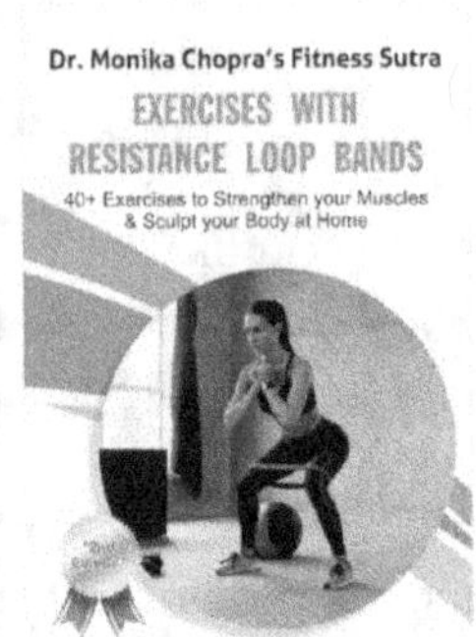

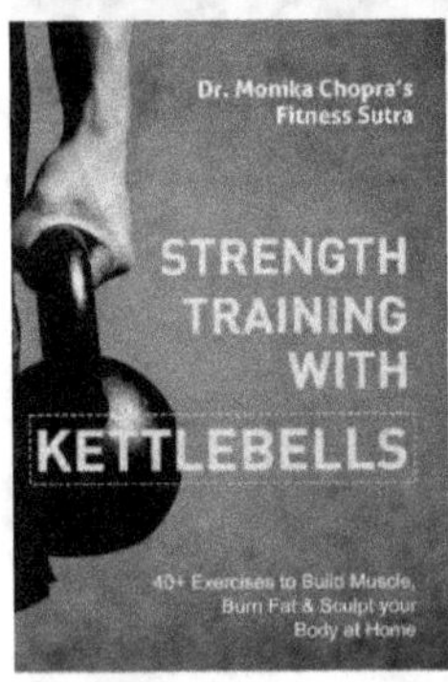


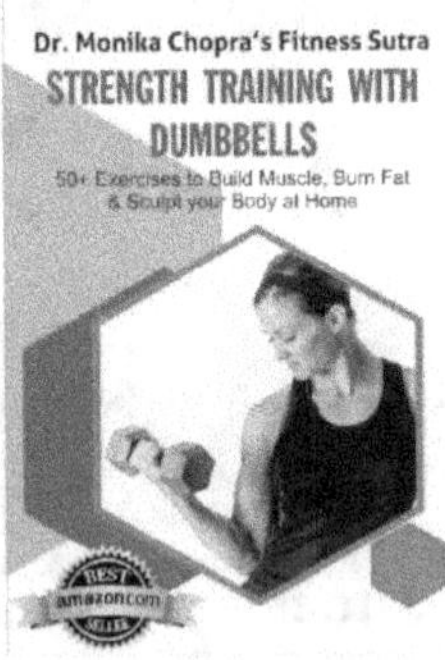


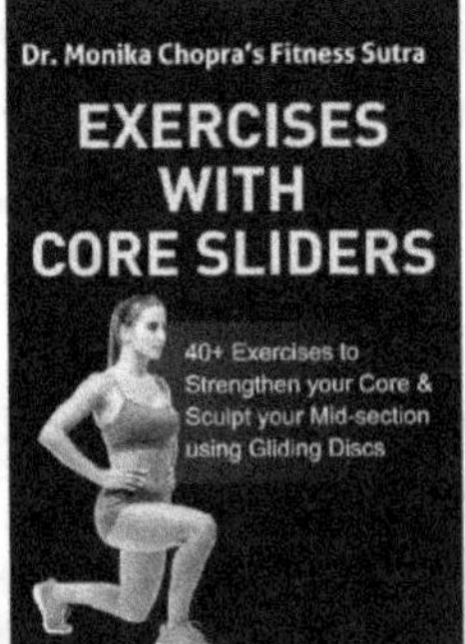


https://www.fitness-sutra.com/go?id=142261